Life After Diabetes

The sudden knowledge that I had diabetes was a cruel shock, similar to the jolt one feels when learning of a loved one's unexpected and untimely death. At first, I felt in denial, but then denial gave way to sadness and a sense of loss and worthlessness. Daily activities seemed futile and exhausting. Slowly, reality checked my bleak thoughts and I knew I had muchmore to live for.

It has been over 28 years since I first developed the disease. Throughout that time, I have enjoyed excellent health, suffering very few common illnesses. With encouragement from my family and friends, I decided that diabetes was not going to incapacitate me, but rather be a unique experience and life-style through which I could make valuable contributions. I hope the reader will find my efforts helpful and, most of all, encouraging.

—Peter A. Lodewick, M.D.

If you have a person with diabetes in the family, this book is a must for your library.

—*Pediatrics for Parents*

A DIABETIC DOCTOR LOOKS AT DIABETES:

His & Yours

Peter A. Lodewick, M.D.

A Newly Revised Edition

A DIABETIC DOCTOR LOOKS AT DIABETES: HIS AND YOURS

Over 85,000 copies sold

New Edition by Gravlee Graphics

ISBN 1890203009

Printed in the United States of America

for Victoria, Peter, Matthew, Sarah
and
for all people concerned with diabetes,
its problems, its solutions,
and its eventual cure.

Contents

Foreword

To the casual observer, *A Diabetic Doctor Looks at Diabetes: His and Yours* might be mistaken for just one more book about diabetes. This would be a serious error. In a field where instructional texts abound, Peter Lodewick now offers a superb and refreshing addition!

The first criterion for any text giving guidelines on the management of diabetes is that it be technically correct and in the mainstream of contemporary thinking. *A Diabetic Doctor Looks at Diabetes: His and Yours* handle this aspect well, but it is the method and style that render it unique and make it a delight to read, rather than a chore.

Dr. Lodewick is able to approach his topic from the dual perspective of both patient and physician. He is not afraid to deal with the emotional issues that challenge all newly diag-nosed person with diabetes or to discuss these frankly and openly. Many real people appear on the pages to follow, and they give the book an added dimension. The case examples run the gamut from poignant to hilarious. Is it possible to face the challenge of managing diabetes without losing your sense of humor? The answer is an emphatic "yes." An ability not only to carry on courageously but to laugh in the face of adversity is a highly desirable gift. When this is mixed with an equal proportion of the desire to live life in the fullest sense, diabetes is not going to be any deterrent to success. As Adam Lindsay Gordon said,

> *Question not but live and labour*
> *Til your goal be won,*
> *Helping every feeble neighbor,*
> *Seeking help from none;*
> *Life is mostly froth and bubble*
> *Two things stand like stone:*
> *Kindness in another's trouble,*
> *Courage in our own.*

Peter Lodewick has an unbeatable attitude and a real ability to laugh at adversity without ignoring the threat. This is the message that abounds on the pages of this book.

In the many years since writing the foreword to the first edition, I have recommended Dr. Lodewick's book to many of my patients, who have commented favorably as they found it both helpful and enjoyable. The revisions in the subsequent editions have further improved this fine book, and I will continue to use it in my own practice.

THOMAS M. FLOOD, M.D.
Medical Director
Georgia Center for Diabetes
Atlanta, Georgia *and*
Past President
American Diabetes Association,
Georgia Affiliate
November 1996

Acknowledgements

I could not have written this book alone and am indebted to many people. Most importantly, I am indebted to my countless patients, who have taught me more about diabetes than I could possibly have learned from reading a textbook. Through them I have come to realize that although there may be such a thing as "Type I diabetes," there is *no such thing* as a "Type I diabetes," for there are as many types of diabetes as there are individuals, and treatment must vary accordingly.

I have special appreciation for the many great hospitals where I have been fortunate enough to work with diabetes, and for the many nurses, physicians, dietitians, CDE's (Diabetes Nurse Educators), and others, both professional and nonprofessional, all over the country who have been a constant source of inspiration.

My thanks to Maureen for her help in reviewing the manuscript of the initial edition of this book.

I am very grateful to Charles A. Thielman, D.P.M., Consultant in Podiatry, a wonderful man and podiatrist, for his help with writing the chapter on foot care; to Elizabeth A. Warholak, R.D., a nutritionist at Zurbrugg Memorial Hospital, for her contribution on the chapter concerning the diabetes diet; and to M. Jeffrey Morton, D.M.D., for writing the chapter on dental care.

My thanks go to Rita Nemchik, R.N., M.S., for her constructive review of the first manuscript. I am also sincerely indebted to Charles A. Suther, for his major contributing efforts in the publication of this book. Anne Waters of RMI reviewed the initial raw manuscript, suggested changes, and transformed my somewhat unclear wording and disjointed sentences into a smooth and readable composition. My appreciation goes also to Amy Troyansky of RMI who enhanced the book considerably with her fine illustrations. I would also like to thank Alison Acker and the family of Bantam Books (former versions) and Srila Sen (1986 version) for their editorial help and enthusiasm on the revised and updated editions.

A special thank you to Jennifer White with Gravlee Graphics for her help and patience in updating and reviewing the manuscript as I prepared for a new edition.

Finally, I would like to thank the new woman in my life, Becky, for all her energy, enthusiasm and **love** she has brought to my life.

A Doctor's Plight

The sudden knowledge that I had diabetes was a cruel shock, similar to the jolt one feels when learning of a loved one's unexpected and untimely death. At first, you are in denial, but then denial gives way to sadness and a sense of loss and worthlessness. Daily activities seem overwhelming and exhausting. Gradually, after a period of grief and idleness, the news becomes a reality that must be confronted, accepted, and integrated into one's life. If I as a doctor considered diabetes so shocking, I cannot imagine how frightening such news must be for a patient.

For me, my newly discovered disease seemed astonishing for several reasons. First of all, I had learned in medical school that diabetes was a hereditary disease. There was no history of diabetes in my family; in fact, all members of my family had enjoyed extraordinarily good health. I cannot recall my parents ever being hospitalized. My four brothers (all within five years of my age) and I had always been exceptionally healthy. We had no healing problems or incidents of recurrent illnesses, two factors known to be associated with diabetes.

Secondly, it was curious that of all the disorders I studied in medical school, the one disease I consciously thought most about and the one I hoped I would never develop was diabetes. I had learned that diabetes often causes high blood pressure, heart disease, gout, kidney disease, gangrene, cataracts, and other visual difficulties. I certainly never wanted a disease that could be so troublesome and that could cause such prolonged suffering. I learned that some people with diabetes had to take insulin injections and that tremendous self-discipline and meticulous care were necessary to maintain good health. During this same period of time, I learned that the younger brother of one of my closest friends had diabetes and that he had to stick to a very strict diet in order to control his disease. From all this, I knew that I definitely did not want diabetes.

The final factor that made me so incredulous about the development of my diabetes was that in my second year of medical school I had learned that my former wife's grandmother had diabetes. Knowing the complications associated with diabetes, I was concerned about Maureen and desperately hoped that she would not become afflicted. It was ironic that I should be the one to develop the disease.

Diabetes is thought to be induced during periods of physical stress (such as surgery or infection) or mental stress anxiety. For me, it was the opposite since it was after my most difficult years that I developed diabetes. During medical school and internship, stress was great. It was troubling to confront very ill people for the first time, hoping to heal them with what seemed to me minimal clinical experience. This stress was compounded by the difficult, vital examinations that had to be passed in order to get my medical degree. My thoughts at these times were - 'What if I should fail? What would I do? What possible work could I find?" And, of course, there were the financial worries that required me to work full time while in medical school and still be thousands of dollars in debt by the time I completed my education. I worked long hours, sometimes without sleeping for 36 hours at a time. My eating habits were poor, and the heavy work schedule prevented me from engaging in daily exercise. Despite the physical and mental stress, however, I felt healthy, productive, and excited about my future.

Following medical school and internship, there was a period of tranquility in my life. I had finished my internship, passed my examination, decided to specialize in ophthalmology, and was assured of a residency program. Before beginning that residency, however, I planned to spend three years in the U.S. Navy as a general medical officer.

During the first few months as a general medical officer, my life was easier and calmer than it had been for years. I was fortunate to be stationed in the United States instead of being sent to the war zone. I had easy hours compared to the rigorous schedule of school and internship. I worked from 8:00 AM to 4:30 PM with a two-hour lunch break. During that lunch break, I resumed a regular exercise program and took up tennis enthusiastically. My responsibilities did not include caring for very sick patients; most of my patients had minor ailments related to colds or skin problems.

My family life was solid and happy. Maureen and I were expecting the birth of our second child. We were in excellent health, and our financial situation was improving. In short, my anxieties had virtually disappeared.

It was during this most tranquil period in my life that diabetes was to manifest itself. Several months after joining the Navy, I had a routine physical examination, and a laboratory technician informed me of a "trace of sugar" in my urine. I was astonished. Certain that he was mistaken, we together retested the specimen using another testing method. This second method (which, we later learned, was **less sensitive than the first**) gave a negative result. No sugar. The thought of potential diabetes completely vanished.

Several months later, I became seriously ill with the Asian flu. My temperature rose to 105 degrees, and I suffered intense headache, backache and nausea. Almost immediately, I started to drink large amounts of water and other fluids, knowing that "fluids help control the fever". And then a baffling thing happened. My fever dissipated, but I still had the urge to drink huge quantities of fluids, especially water. I had never before had such a desire and had seldom drunk more than one full glass of water per day. Even in my beer-drinking days at college, I had not mastered the art of "guzzling," and here I was guzzling, not beer, but plain, tasteless, spiritless water at an enormous rate. Along with my insatiable thirst, my urinary flow increased markedly. Instead of my usual two to three trips per day to the bathroom, I was going six to ten times per day, including several nighttime visits.

Despite these alarming symptoms and my knowledge of their association with diabetes, I was convinced the signs were psychogenic. "After all," I told myself repeatedly, "I'm healthy, I feel good, I've always been healthy. I've rarely been sick, and the same goes for the rest of my family, including my parents and brothers. There was no history of diabetes in the family." I even related my symptoms to my medical colleagues so they could share the absurdity of the situation.

I continued to shrug it off for the next several weeks until some premonition made me get on the scale. My customary "skinny" weight of 162 pounds ("Bones" was a common nickname) had dropped dramatically to an even skinnier 151 pounds. I then decided that it was time to check my urine for sugar. Yes, sugar was present. What had been so laughable suddenly became a source of anguish and depression.

In an attempt to cheer myself, I denied that I had diabetes. I ran two miles daily with the hope of lowering my blood sugar level. Not only were these attempts unsuccessful, but I developed excruciatingly painful "charlie horses" in my leg muscles. (These "charlie horses" frequently accompany uncontrolled diabetes.) Still, I continued to deny that I had diabetes. Finally, one of my colleagues performed a glucose tolerance test on me. The values exceeded 600 mg%, the normal being less than 120 mg%. I attempted further exercise, but with no luck. The common sense approach I used with my patients didn't seem to apply to me.

With the gentle urging of Maureen, my family and friends, I gradually overcame my reluctance to be hospitalized. There I was, dazed that I should be in the hospital, unable to come to grips with my ill fortune. I wrongfully assumed that I would soon be incapacitated by all the ailments I had studied in my years of medical training and that I would not be able to care for my wife and children. I doubted whether I would be able to complete my term in the Navy or finish my planned ophthalmology residency.

Slowly, reality checked my bleak thoughts. How foolish could I be? "Physician, heal thyself." With encouragement from my family and friends, I decided that diabetes was not going to incapacitate me but rather be a unique experience and lifestyle through which I could make valuable contributions.

Four years after the discovery of my diabetes, much had changed. I decided that instead of serving as a general medical officer, I would begin my residency in the Navy. During that residency, I decided to study internal medicine and diabetes rather than ophthalmology.

Much to my dismay, I was not able to continue in the Navy because of my diabetes. This disappointment was not long-lasting, however, for I was able to study internal medicine and diabetes under dedicated physicians at the Joslin Clinic who had some 30 to 50 years of experience in the field. I also had the opportunity to supervise a large children's diabetes camp, where I became convinced that diabetes did not prevent children from living full, active lives.

The initial shock and fears I had when I first discovered my diabetes rapidly wore off. All the complications I initially dreaded have not developed in over 28 years of living with diabetes. I have not missed one day of work despite working many 24-hour days in the practice of medicine. Throughout that time, I have enjoyed excellent health, and suffered very few common illnesses. I have four children, ages 29, 27, 25 and our youngest who is 17—all of whom are very healthy young adults.

I jog long distances and, as you will learn throughout this book, I play unbeatable tennis. Yes, it is possible that I will develop some of the complications I feared so much in medical school, but those thoughts are rare because I have so many exciting challenges that are with me as I greet each day.

Yes, I have to take insulin shots. However, were it not for the discovery of insulin in 1921, my chances of survival would have been slim. I am both amazed and thankful, viewing insulin as a miracle drug that gives me strength and vigor. This attitude toward insulin injection helps me accept this minor inconvenience in my daily life—at least until diabetes research comes up with something else, which I truly think will be the case given the tremendous advancements that have already been made.

Now, I use my experience with diabetes to help others cope, understand, and live with diabetes healthily. I have found over the last 28 years, I can fulfill all of my dreams even if I have diabetes. One of those dreams being to write books. I have authored this book and co-authored another called, *The Diabetic Man*. Who knows what else I find I can achieve.

The information in this book I have gathered from my personal experience with diabetes, from my practice as a physician working with person with diabetes and from the expertise I've observed from other physicians in the field of diabetes. I hope the reader will find my efforts helpful and, most of all, encouraging.

– Peter A. Lodewick, M.D.
November, 1996

Dr. Lodewick's Profile

Age: 54

Age of Diabetes Onset: 26 years [Year Diagnosed: 1968]

Duration: 28 years

Health Status: No major complications

		Normal Values
Blood Pressure:	138/82 mm HG	< 140/85 mm HG
Electrocardiogram:	Normal	
Total Cholesterol:	180mg%	Less than 200mg%
HDL Cholesterol:	61mg%	Over 40mg%
LDL Cholesterol:	117mg%	Under 160mg%
Triglycerides:	44mg%	Under 150mg%
Average Fasting Blood Sugar:	140mg%	Under 100mg%
Glycohemoglobin:	8.3%	4.4 to 8.2 percent
Urine Protein:	Negative	Negative

Family History: Negative for diabetes in large family

Exercise: Jogs 3 to 6 miles a day, 3 to 5 times a week [Total of 14 to 20 miles a week; 750 to 900 miles a year; topped 1000 miles in 1991] Tennis: "Outplay most high school tennis players."

Diet: 2000 to 2400 Calories per day. Low fat intake; Drinks distilled water.

Physical Exam: Once a year

Eye Exam: Once a year [Has no evidence of retinopathy, 1996]

Stress Electrocardiogram: Every 5 years; no evidence of heart disease following Thallium test in 1993

Work: Full-time physician and diabetes specialist

Hobbies: Writing, reading, tennis, gardening and my family life

Dr. Lodewick has had diabetes for over 28 years. As you can see, this has not slowed him down. As Dr. Lodewick says;
"I feel lucky that I have been in the medical field, and have had first hand experience with diabetes-related problems and how to avoid these problems. I hope that you, the reader, will learn the needed material to prevent diabetes from slowing you down — at least until science and medicine can develop better treatment methods and one day find the ultimate cure."

1

What Is Diabetes?

The only defense against the world is a thorough knowledge of it.
                                                    -JOHN LOCKE

There are millions of people in the United States who have
diabetes. For these people, knowledge about the disease and
how it is controlled is a prerequisite to proper self management. In this world of instant communication, I would think
that the people who need to know the most about diabetes
would have very easy access to helpful information.
However, as a practicing diabetes specialist I am constantly
astonished by the number of patients who are totally in the
dark about the disease that afflicts so many. This is true not
only for people with diabetes, but also for their families,
friends and even some of the doctors and nurses who treat
them.

What Is Sugar?

Many people are surprised to learn that sugar is as necessary for the person with diabetes as well as the person without diabetes, since it fuels many basic functions of the body. I
have often heard the exclamation, "He's diabetic and he's eating sugar!" There is some validity to this accusation, but only
if the person with diabetes has very high blood sugars and
poor control of the disease. It must
be emphasized, however, that the person with diabetes *does*
need sugar just as the non-diabetic does. The problem is how
to *maintain* as excellent control of blood sugar levels as the
non-diabetic.

Sugar is the simplest form of carbohydrate and is the

1

body's major energy source for sustaining life. Body cells need approximately 100 to 300 or more grams (20 to 60 teaspoons) of sugar per day. It is the major calorie source for the brain! And without it the brain cannot function.

When we talk about blood sugar, we actually mean blood glucose, which is a specific form of simple sugar required by the body cells as an energy source. There are several types of sugar, all of which are forms of carbohydrates and all of which can be converted to glucose. These sugars include table sugar, milk sugar (lactose), fruit sugar (fructose), as well as the more complex sugar forms found in vegetables, breads, and starches. Glucose can be made from about 60% of the protein and 10% of the fat in our diet. Thus, a wide variety of foods, not just simple sugars, can raise blood sugar levels in people with diabetes.

Besides being the major energy source for all cells, simple sugar or glucose (these words will be used interchangeably throughout this book) is thought to be the only energy source for brain and nerve cells. In short, without glucose we cannot live.

When a person without diabetes consumes food, the simple and complex carbohydrates contained in the food are converted to glucose, causing a slight rise in blood glucose levels. These elevated glucose levels trigger the release of the hormone *insulin* from a gland in the abdomen called the *pancreas*. Insulin regulates the amount of glucose in the bloodstream and facilitates utilization of this glucose as an energy source by cells. When more food is consumed than is immediately necessary, excess glucose is converted into another form of sugar called glycogen, which is stored in muscles and the liver for future energy needs. Without insulin, glucose cannot be properly utilized or stored.

In diabetes, there is a dysfunction in one of two mechanisms: either there is a deficiency or a complete absence in insulin production, or body cells are unable to use the insulin properly. Thus, glucose cannot be escorted properly into body cells for energy production. The unused glucose accumulates in the blood and spills into the urine. The high glucose levels may be responsible for many medical complications that are associated with diabetes.

Before going any further, it is important to understand that diabetes is not just a simple problem of "too much sugar." Insulin also has an effect on muscle and fat metabolism, facilitating protein and fat synthesis. Thus, when insulin is deficient or the cells are not using it properly, not only does the blood sugar build up, but if this process is unchecked (as in uncontrolled diabetes), the body breaks down fat and protein in its attempt to provide energy. This breakdown of fat and protein forms acidic toxins, resulting in acidosis or ketosis, which can be life threatening (see Chapter 10, "Low and High Blood Sugar Reactions: Hypoglycemia and Ketoacidosis").

The Discovery of Insulin

For many centuries, we knew very little about the cause of diabetes, although the characteristic signs and symptoms were well described. Some patients were known to experience a very rapid onset of symptoms, including unquenchable thirst, excessive urination, dry skin and mouth, and massive weight loss that made them look starved. For many people, particularly children, several modes of partially effective treatments were attempted to alleviate this dire chain of events, but ultimately death followed.

In the early part of the twentieth century, it became apparent that food and diet played a significant role in diabetes; carbohydrates were known especially to aggravate the disease. High-fat diets were tried but did little good. In many cases, the only way to keep people with diabetes alive was with a minimal amount of calories (sometimes as low as 400 calories per day) and with alcohol, which provided a ready source of energy not requiring insulin. Even then, the patient remained extremely ill and could barely leave the house since any form of exercise made his condition worse. This sort of life-style was indeed a dismal one and for most people with this type of diabetes, death would follow.

Finally, in the 1920s, insulin was discovered through the diligent efforts of Drs. Frederick G. Banting and Charles H. Best. Thanks to their persistent research, insulin was identified as the substance that was deficient or absent in many people with diabetes, making them unable to utilize glucose properly. It has since been discovered that insulin is secreted by a small group of cells in the pancreas, called the *beta cells*. Surprisingly, the beta cells comprise less than one percent of the total number of cells that make up the pancreas. The majority of the cells of the pancreas are used to help digest protein, fat, and carbohydrate in the small intestine, but it is the beta cells, with less than a total weight of 1 to 2 ounces, which provide all the insulin required to keep the blood glucose levels within the normal range of about 60-to-120mg% (which means that there is about one teaspoon of glucose in the blood at any given time) and allow the cells to utilize the glucose properly. It is amazing that in non-diabetics these
beta cells, which make up such a small part of the pancreas, can continue to function so effectively despite the fact that they are continuously barraged by tremendous amounts of carbohydrate (up to 60 or more teaspoons of sugar or carbohydrate equivalent per day). In diabetes this delicate beta cell mechanism fails, as I will discuss in detail in some of the following chapters.

2

Types of Diabetes

Type I Insulin-Dependent Diabetes

After the discovery of insulin by Banting and Best, it was thought that all types of diabetes were caused by the failure of beta cells to produce insulin. Since then, however, research has proven this to be only partially true. Probably less than 20% of people with diabetes have the type of diabetes in which the beta cells fail to produce insulin. This type of diabetes is now called *Type I insulin-dependent diabetes* because insulin, administered by injection, is needed to control the disease. It should also be understood that even in this type of diabetes, there are various levels of beta cell failure. In some insulin-dependent diabetes, insulin produced by the beta cells is just not enough. The different degrees of beta cell failure that occur among Type I insulin-dependent diabetes may partially explain the fact that each patient requires individualized amounts of insulin to control their disease.

Although we know that the failure of the beta cells to produce insulin is responsible for Type I insulin-dependent diabetes, it is still a mystery as to why the beta cells fail in the first place (see Chapter 30, "Research—Quest for a Cure" for more information). It is speculated that these cells may have been attacked by the viruses that cause mumps, infectious mononucleosis, influenza or rubella; by the Coxsackie virus; or other viruses; or by beta cell antibodies that may suddenly be produced by the body for an unknown reason. Because of the antibodies that are produced by the person's own body, this disease is now considered one of the "autoimmune diseases." There are many of these autoimmune diseases, including several of the glandular organs, such as the thyroid and sexual organs. Genetic and psychological factors may also affect the beta cells and make them unable to function properly. Excessive food or sugar intake does not contribute to the development of insulin-dependent diabetes. However, once the disease has developed, it is believed that excessive food or sugar will stress the beta cell reserve and make the diabetes more difficult to control.

Type II Non-Insulin-Dependent Diabetes

In contrast to the insulin-dependent diabetes, the majority of people with diabetes (possibly more than 80%) do produce certain amounts of insulin, but not quite enough to keep the blood sugar normal. In fact, in the 1960s Dr. Jesse Roth, a researcher with the National Institutes of Health, made the tremendous discovery that many people with diabetes produce at least normal or higher than normal amounts of insulin. This may sound confusing, since it would seem that diabetes would not exist if normal amounts of insulin are produced. However, research stemming from Dr. Roth's work has shown that diabetes occurs in the presence of normal or higher insulin levels because in this type of diabetes the insulin does not function effectively. For insulin to be effective, it must attach itself to the different body cells (such as muscle, liver, fat, or white blood cells) at *receptor sites*. If the receptor sites are defective or if there are not enough of them, then the cells do not accept the insulin *(insulin resistance)* When this occurs, insulin does not function properly and does

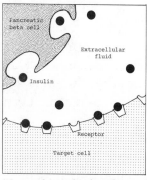

Normal insulin level.

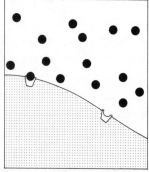

Increased insulin level due to fewer receptor sites, as in Type II diabetes.

not escort glucose into the cells and blood glucose levels rise. Since insulin is present in normal or elevated amounts in this type of diabetes, insulin injections are not usually needed. This form of diabetes is now referred to as *Type II non-insulin-dependent diabetes.*

Other Distinctions Between Type I Insulin-Dependent and Type II Non-Insulin-Dependent Diabetes

Another difference between Type I insulin-dependent and Type II non-insulin-dependent diabetes relates to average age of onset. The insulin-dependent form was originally called juvenile diabetes since it typically occurred in people under the age of 25. In contrast, the non-insulin dependent type was frequently referred to as "adult-onset diabetes" because it had a tendency to occur in people over the age of 30.

There are important exceptions to this "adult-onset" vs. "juvenile onset" terminology, however. Insulin-dependent diabetes *can* occur in middle or late adulthood, and conversely, recent studies have pointed to cases of non-insulin-dependent diabetes that have occurred in youths under the age of 20. Given these exceptions, "insulin-dependent" is *not* identical to "juvenile-onset," nor is "non-insulin-dependent" identical to "adult-onset." However, in a large percentage of cases, age of onset is often an indication of whether or not the patient will need insulin.

Another major difference between Type I insulin-dependent and Type II non-insulin-dependent diabetes involves the degree of glucose fluctuation. In Type II non-insulin-dependent diabetes, the blood glucose level may run as high as 320mg%, but it may not vary much throughout the day; it may be 320mg% in the morning, 330mg% at noon, and 300mg% in the evening. It seems that glucose levels are not affected greatly by daily changes of food intake or activity. In contrast, there can be marked fluctuations in blood glucose levels for some Type I insulin-dependent people with diabetes despite very little variation in activity or diet. Levels can go from 60mg% up to 600mg% and back to 50mg% all in the same day.

A final difference that I would like to mention concerns heredity. There tends to be a hereditary link among people with Type II non-insulin-dependent diabetes. There may be as many as six brothers or sisters all of whom have non-insulin-dependent diabetes. This hereditary pattern is much less apparent in insulin-dependent diabetes. A child may develop insulin-dependent diabetes when there is absolutely no family history of the disease. Again, there are exceptions. I have seen several families in my own practice where two or more children developed insulin-dependent diabetes under the age of 10. Thus, it is apparent that heredity, age, glucose level fluctu-

Insulin-Dependent vs. Non-Insulin-Dependent Diabetes

	Type I Insulin-Dependent	Type II Non-Insulin Dependent
Age of Onset	Usually less than 20 years, but can be any age	Usually over 30 years, but a small number of cases develop the disease before the age of 30
"Tip-Off"	Abrupt onset of symptoms with weight loss	Slow onset of symptoms, sometimes with weight gain
Family History	At first, may be none, but as years pass, family history may manifest itself as a factor	Commonly a factor
Stability	Not very stable; must closely monitor changes in insulin, exercise, and food intake, which affect blood sugar markedly	More stable; changes in insulin, exercise, and food have much less dramatic effect on blood sugar
Control of Diabetes	Difficult	Less Difficult
Complications	May occur	May occur
Diet	Vitally important	Important, and may determine whether or not patient needs insulin or pills
Insulin Need	Yes—100%	Needed in only 20-30% of cases
Need for Pills	No	Sometimes

ation, and many other factors seem to have some correlation to the type of diabetes that develops, but there are no hard and fast rules at this point in our understanding of diabetes.

On the previous page is a summary chart that highlights the major differences between insulin-dependent and non-insulin-dependent diabetes.

Besides the differentiation between Type I insulin-dependent and Type II non-insulin-dependent diabetes, there are other terms that come up frequently when diabetes is discussed. These terms are discussed below.

Prediabetes

Pre-diabetes has been used to describe a person who is basically healthy but who will eventually develop diabetes. The problem is that there is still no way of predicting accurately who will develop diabetes. The chances are much higher in children whose parents both have diabetes, or in the identical twin of a person with diabetes, but even here there is no perfect correlation. Individuals who have strong family histories of diabetes are being studied very closely in many centers around the world in an effort to pinpoint the predisposing factors of diabetes and to uncover the actual cause of the disease.

Chemical Diabetes or Impaired Glucose Tolerance or "Borderline Diabetes"

Chemical diabetes refers to a condition in which blood glucose abnormality or "glucose intolerance" is confirmed by laboratory tests but overt diabetes symptoms are not present. There are two stages of chemical diabetes: latent and pure. In *latent chemical diabetes,* the glucose intolerance (or abnormal blood sugar) is induced by stress, pregnancy, drugs, surgery, or infection, but the glucose intolerance disappears under more normal basal conditions. Latent diabetes may progress to another stage, *pure chemical diabetes,* in which blood sugar is elevated after fasting. This is sometimes referred to as

"Borderline Diabetes". However, this condition should not be taken lightly. In combination with high blood pressure and high cholesterol, it can be associated with many medical problems. Also, it is more important that individuals with these forms of glucose intolerance avoid overeating, obesity, and certain medicines (unless recommended by a physician) because these forms of diabetes can progress to overt diabetes. Then again, I have seen some patients with chemical diabetes who have participated in studies for up to 50 years and who have had *none* of the complications that are normally seen in overt diabetes. Exceptions, exceptions!

Overt Diabetes

Overt diabetes refers to the symptomatic onset of diabetes. Many cases of overt diabetes are not known to have been preceded by glucose intolerance. These cases are often characterized by abrupt onset with frequent urination, excess hunger and thirst, and weight loss. Sometimes (especially in very young children) these symptoms may be present for only one to two days before diabetes coma develops. These cases are especially typical of insulin-dependent Type I diabetes.

In contrast, the symptoms of Type II diabetes may be very subtle, or may even have no symptoms, and the patient may have diabetes for many years without knowing it. Type II diabetes is usually associated with obesity, fatigue, increased urination and excessive thirst. Some with Type II diabetes will have a rather abrupt onset more characteristic of Type I and may in fact become insulin-dependent. Any one who has a family history of diabetes should know about the characteristic symptoms of this disease (see Chapter 4, "Subtle Signs of Diabetes" for more information). With this knowledge, primary or hereditary diabetes can be diagnosed and treated earlier, possibly resulting in fewer complications.

Secondary Diabetes (Glucose Intolerance Associated with Other Conditions)

Secondary diabetes is a type of diabetes induced by other conditions or disorders. The most obvious example is diabetes induced by surgical removal of the pancreas or by destruction of pancreatic tissue due to tumor, inflammation, or infection. In addition, there are several other disorders that affect body metabolism in such a way that diabetes can develop. These disorders include overactive thyroid gland, overactive pituitary gland (producing too much growth hormone) and overactive adrenal gland (producing too much cortisol or adrenaline). Proper treatment of these underlying endocrine disorders usually causes diabetes symptoms to disappear unless the patient has underlying primary diabetes as well. Other conditions that may induce diabetes include excessive or prolonged use of alcohol, malnutrition and the use of certain pills, especially birth control pills, water pills (diuretics), diet pills and several other medications. Obviously, not all people who drink excessive alcohol or use pills will develop diabetes. The point is that those with an *underlying predisposition* may develop diabetes symptoms that often disappear with abstention from alcohol and the above-mentioned drugs.

3

The Natural Course of Diabetes

As you will discover, the course of diabetes is a winding one, and no two cases will be alike. Each person with diabetes has a unique personality, physique, metabolism, and attitude toward diet, exercise, and life in general. Since these factors influence diabetes, the course of the disease will vary with the individual. In some respects, the person with diabetes must be his own doctor, for it is impossible for his physician to understand all the moods, activities and social situations that will affect him. The more the person with diabetes knows about himself, about diabetes, and about the interrelationships of diet, food, exercise, moods and blood sugar, the more he will be able to direct the course of his condition to live many years without complications.

Autoimmunity factors that precipitate diabetes have not yet been isolated; however, heredity, viruses, infections, and emotional problems have all been implicated. The fact that the onset of diabetes can occur at ages ranging from 6 months to 68 years is still puzzling. Without an easy explanation for the onset of diabetes, the development of the disease is usually a shock to most people. For older people accustomed to good health, they find it hard to believe that diabetes can suddenly present itself. Unfortunately, because some people deny that they have diabetes, they fail to learn basic information that can benefit them enormously. By learning about these complications, the person with diabetes may be much more motivated to learn how to avoid them.

Course of Insulin-Dependent Diabetes

Type I insulin-dependent diabetes usually presents itself with intense symptoms of thirst, excessive urination, dry

12

mouth, loss of energy, fatigue, weight loss, muscle cramps, and blood sugars over 300mg%. If diabetes is not diagnosed soon enough, these symptoms can progress to diabetes coma or ketoacidosis (see Chapter 10, "Low and High Blood Sugar Reactions: Hypoglycemia and Ketoacidosis" for more information). Type I insulin-dependent diabetes occurs most commonly in younger people, but I have seen exceptions where it has occurred in people in their seventies. In most cases, the symptoms are present for three months or less prior to diagnosis. Occasionally, the symptoms can be so severe that they progress to coma within 24 hours, the patient having had no apparent symptoms a day earlier.

Once the diagnosis is made, diet and insulin injections are needed, and the symptoms rapidly disappear. Diabetes may then go into what is called a "remission" or "honeymoon" phase, where symptoms level off. The more overweight the person, the more likely that remission will occur. It can also occur in children. During remission, the pancreas secretes insulin again and the need for insulin injections decreases and may actually disappear for a time.

During a phase of remission, persons with diabetes frequently have trouble believing that they do in fact have diabetes. It is not uncommon for the patient, or parents of a child with diabetes, to wonder whether the diagnosis might have been mistaken and, understandably, to hope that it was. For a while, their hope may seem justified as blood sugars remain near normal. However, the period of remission ends (generally within two years but occasionally after a longer period) and blood sugar again goes up, requiring increased amounts of insulin. What terminates the remission phase is as little understood as what causes diabetes to occur in the first place, but factors such as poor diet, acute infections, growth of the patient and body changes related to adolescence are thought to be part of the cause.

Emphasis should be placed on the critical factor of food intake. Although diet has nothing to do with causing this type of diabetes, it has a major effect on the remission phase. Over and over again, I have seen cases in which overeating has exacerbated the underlying tendency toward diabetes and shortened the period of remission. Therefore, it is very important to plan the diet carefully, with the goal to maintain ideal weight and maximum strength without over- or under-eating.

As the remission phase ends, the diabetes becomes less stable as the pancreas secret varying amounts of insulin, and insulin injection may again be needed in increasing amounts. The diabetes may then develop into what is called "brittle diabetes," in which blood sugars can fluctuate from 100mg% to 600mg% and back to 100mg% all in the same day with little change in activity, insulin, or exercise (See Chapter 11, "The Effects of Insulin Over-Use: Brittle Diabetes and The Somogyi Effect").

In the course of insulin-dependent diabetes, certain associated medical problems may occur; however, it must be emphasized that many of them are avoidable. The two major conditions that can usually be prevented are ketoacidosis and hypoglycemia, both of which could lead to a diabetes coma if left untreated. These conditions will be discussed in more detail in Chapter 10, "Low and High Blood Sugar Reactions: Hypoglycemia and Ketoacidosis," but some introductory points should be made here.

Ketoacidosis results from a lack of insulin, which causes elevated blood sugars and breakdown of fat into dangerous ketoacid bodies. I have seen patients hospitalized repeatedly with this potentially fatal condition and cannot understand why they let it happen. Ketoacidosis may be caused by omission of the patient's usual insulin dose, by overeating, or by a major illness such as pneumonia or kidney infection. Often, the patient simply does not know he has diabetes and therefore does not recognize the symptoms or know how to prevent their progression to coma. In practically every case, ketoacidosis can be prevented if care is taken.

The other type of diabetes coma, hypoglycemia, or low blood sugar (usually less than 40mg%), results from too much insulin, excessive exercise or too little food. It is my experience that most cases of this type of coma are also completely avoidable. Most of the cases I have seen occurred in people who did not have adequate knowledge of insulin, food, exercise, or their interaction and did not use urine testing or blood sugar testing as a guide to controlling their blood sugars. It is reassuring to know that most cases of hypoglycemia are mild and easily reversible, and even the more severe ones do not cause permanent damage. However, they are unpleasant and can be embarrassing.

Long-term complications associated with insulin-dependent diabetes can be: loss of vision due to bleeding in the eye, from retinopathy, heart disease, neuropathy, neuritis, impotence, kidney disease and blood vessel disease of the legs that causes increased susceptibility to infection and gangrene of the legs and feet. Cataract formation does not necessarily occur in a greater percentage of people with diabetes than of the general population, but it tends to occur at an earlier age. Up to eight percent of people with insulin dependent diabetes lose vision as a result of their disease. However, as discussed in the section on complications, most of these complications can be prevented by good care.

At present, heart disease is the primary cause of poor health in people with diabetes. Elevated blood sugars and lack of exercise, along with poor diet, are in my opinion factors that accelerate heart disease in people with diabetes. As will be discussed later in the dietary chapter, Chapter 13, "The Diabetic Diet—Food, Glorious Food."

Despite the prevalence of the foregoing complications, not all insulin-dependent diabetes will develop them. Many of these diabetes have lived over 50 years without suffering any of the major complications. In fact, the Joslin Diabetes Center in Boston, the largest center in the world for the study and treatment of diabetes, gives awards to patients who have had diabetes for over 50 years. They have given this award to hundreds of patients with diabetes. It *can* be done!

Course of Type II Non-Insulin-Dependent Diabetes

The course of Type II non-insulin-dependent diabetes is somewhat different from that of insulin-dependent diabetes.

Since the onset is not as acute and blood sugars are not as high, a person with diabetes may tolerate symptoms for a long time, thus delaying diagnosis. Because the symptoms are hard to pinpoint (see Chapter 4, "Subtle Signs of Diabetes"), it is possible for years to pass before the diagnosis is made. Some of the symptoms include fatigue, which the patient may attribute to "just getting older," and weight gain, passed off as "middle-age spread." The increased thirst associated with high blood sugar becomes so constant that the patient may consider it normal, stating, "I've always been thirsty." Finally (often at the urging of a spouse), the patient has a medical checkup, and the diagnosis is made. Unfortunately, when diabetes has already been present for some time, complications may also be present at diagnosis. It is not uncommon, for instance, to find indications of heart disease, vascular disease, impotence, or small blood vessel disease at the time of diagnosis.

At this point, I would like to reassure you that the diagnosis of diabetes does not mean instant defeat necessitating a total change in lifestyle. The majority of people diagnosed with diabetes will never have any of the major complications that are attributed directly to diabetes, particularly if they take the precautions recommended by their physicians with regard to diet, exercise, and preventive care. This is particularly the case with newly diagnosed diabetes who are over the age of 50.

The other good news for the person with Type II non-insulin-dependent diabetes is that blood sugars can frequently be controlled with proper diet (probably the most critical factor in control), exercise and possibly diabetes pills, so that insulin is not needed. Unlike the remission phase in Type I insulin-dependent diabetes, which is usually temporary, remissions in Type II non-insulin dependent diabetes can be permanent. Blood sugars may return to normal and stay that way—especially if good diet and exercise are maintained.

A major complication, ketoacidosis, is unlikely since it occurs with insulin deficiency, a condition not present in adult-onset, non-insulin-dependent diabetes. Also, since most people with Type II diabetes do not use insulin, hypoglycemic or low blood sugar-induced coma is not as common, although it can occur with those who are taking diabetes pills.

4

Subtle Signs of Diabetes

As a physician, one question I am repeatedly asked is: Are there any warning signs that indicate that diabetes may be present or that it will develop? People frequently ask this question out of concern for their children or other family members. The answer to this question is that anyone with a family history or with any of the typical symptoms of diabetes or insulin deficiency (such as thirst, excessive urination, weight loss), as discussed in the preceding chapters, should be checked for diabetes. In addition, there are many more subtle signs or symptoms that may indicate the presence of diabetes. Some of these signs and symptoms are discussed below.

Skin Changes

Infections or skin changes are often the initial sign of diabetes, probably occurring in over 25% of people with diabetes who have poor control of their disease. Boils or skin abscesses are bacterial infections that may become severe in a person with diabetes. If untreated, these boils can spread internally and have serious consequences.

Fungal infections may also point to diabetes. Again, these infections are very common in poorly controlled diabetes. If the fungal infection becomes severe enough, it may cause "breaks" in the skin, which can then become infected with bacteria. *Candida* or *Monilia* yeast is one of the most common types of infections in the person with diabetes because this fungus seems to thrive in a high-sugar environment. Presence of this yeast is evidenced by redness, itching, and malodor. Because the yeast prefers moist areas of the body, common sites of infection include the feet, vagina and genital areas. Unless the diabetes is better controlled these infections are difficult to treat.

Another skin lesion that signals diabetes is the "shin spot," a brown, round area about the size of a dime. Occurring particularly on the leg, it is thought that incidental bangs on the shins cause them, but this explanation has not been proven.

Other changes in the skin that may indicate diabetes include loss of hair and loss of sweat glands (so that the skin becomes dry). The skin typically becomes thickened and discolored, and sometimes the nails become thickened as well. Doctors believe that the cause of these changes is probably small blood vessel disease and/or nerve disease (neuropathy), which prevents the skin from getting adequate nourishment. For more information on how to protect and care for the skin, see Chapter 21, "Care of the Skin."

Pregnancy

Diabetes often manifests itself during pregnancy, as discussed more fully in Chapter 23, "Diabetes and the Woman: The Menses, Sexual Response and Pregnancy." As pregnancy progresses, blood sugar levels can become elevated, resulting in "pregnancy diabetes." This form of diabetes often disappears (sometimes only temporarily) following the pregnancy. Because of this tendency for pregnancy to trigger a form of diabetes, I certainly recommend that blood sugars be checked every six weeks or so during the pregnancy, especially if the woman has a family history of diabetes. Then, if the blood sugar level does get high, measures can be taken to assure more normal blood sugars and a more successful pregnancy.

Two other characteristics of a pregnancy that may signal the development of diabetes in the mother include the birth of a heavy baby (over 10 pounds) and premature delivery. It is estimated that up to 20% of the mothers who have large babies will develop diabetes. It is speculated that the extra weight of the baby may actually be caused by high blood sugar levels in the pregnant mother. High blood sugar levels in the mother cause increased insulin secretion by the pancreas of the fetus. This excessive fetal insulin secretion causes extra growth of body tissue in the baby The connection between premature delivery and diabetes is not yet fully understood, but a possible association has been observed.

Obesity

Although not all obese people develop diabetes, those with a genetic predisposition to the disease are taking a much bigger risk of developing it by overeating and accumulating excessive weight. Overeating and obesity trigger increased insulin secretion from the pancreas, resulting in the additional storage of fat in the tissues. As weight and, thereby insulin secretion goes up, the body eventually develops a resistance to the effects of insulin, and diabetes occurs. This course of events represents the typical Type II non-insulin-dependent pattern of diabetes. If the diabetes is poorly controlled for an extended time period, it is my hunch that insulin reserves can become depleted to such a degree that the non-insulin dependent person with diabetes can become insulin-dependent.

Hypoglycemia

Another possible sign of diabetes, which frequently occurs in the obese person, is hypoglycemia, or low blood sugar (usually under 50mg%). As discussed below, there are other conditions that can cause hypoglycemia or hypoglycemic symptoms that have nothing to do with diabetes. But when hypoglycemia is an early indication of diabetes, it usually occurs several hours after a meal, particularly a meal high in simple sugars. Upon eating such a meal, there is a sluggish release of insulin from the pancreas so that initial blood sugars may be high. Several hours later, however, when food has already been absorbed and assimilated, the blood sugar levels may drop below 50mg% as blood insulin levels reach their peak. The blood sugar response to ingested food might be

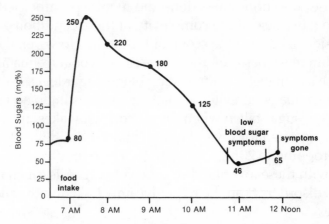

similar to the blood sugar levels shown in the following graph.

As you can see from this graph, low blood sugar symptoms usually occur when the blood sugar falls below 50mg%. These symptoms may include hunger, nervousness, sweating, faintness, irritability and (rarely) loss of consciousness. These symptoms are usually relieved by food, especially sugar foods, but they frequently disappear even without eating food since blood sugar levels tend to normalize due to the increased levels of hormones (adrenaline and glucagon) in the blood, which occur in response to falling blood sugars. In fact, the increased level of hormones, especially adrenaline, may be the actual cause of some of these symptoms.

Although this type of hypoglycemia can be a sign of early diabetes, less than 20% of the people who experience this type of low blood sugar will develop diabetes. Nevertheless, the possibility of diabetes should be explored. A well-balanced, low-sugar, high-fiber, high-carbohydrate diet should prevent the symptoms associated with this hypoglycemia.

Causes of Hypoglycemia Not Related to Diabetes

As mentioned above, it is important to recognize that there are other causes of hypoglycemia that have nothing to do with diabetes. These causes include starvation, alcoholism, underactive adrenal or pituitary glands, liver disease (cirrhosis or hepatitis), drugs, cancer and tumors of the beta cells (causing the cells to produce excessive insulin).

These conditions are serious and require prompt medical attention. Because of the complexity of these conditions, a full discussion is beyond the scope of this book. However, the main difference between these causes of hypoglycemia and that of early diabetes is the fasting blood sugar level. If the hypoglycemia is unrelated to diabetes, the fasting blood sugar (the blood sugar taken when the person just wakes up after not having eaten for several hours) may be less than 50mg%, even dropping to 20mg% or 30mg%. The hypoglycemia associated with these low blood sugar levels suggests much more serious disorders than the hypoglycemia linked with mild diabetes.

When Hypoglycemia is Not Hypoglycemia

In my medical practice I have seen many cases in which people with symptoms of nervousness, shakes, faintness, palpitations, sweats, irritability, depression and fatigue have been diagnosed as having hypoglycemia. Reviewing the symptoms of these individuals, however, it is apparent that the pattern of these symptoms is different from the pattern associated with the hypoglycemia in mild diabetes or the hypoglycemia due to more serious disorders. In comparison with truly hypoglycemic patients, these people have symptoms that appear very suddenly and have little relation to food or sugar intake. They may occur in the morning before food is eaten and then last for hours or days. Upon laboratory analysis, however, these people have blood sugar levels between 60mg% and 100mg%—normal blood sugars! Some people may insist that a value of 66mg% for blood sugar is low (for some, it is relatively low since they get symptomatic from this level, especially if they are used to levels above 200mg%, but this value is within the normal range. It is my strong contention that it is far better to have blood sugars in the 50-to-100mg% range than it is to have levels above 100mg% that may indicate diabetes).

If these people do not have hypoglycemia, then what do they have? There are several conditions that can cause symptoms similar to those caused by hypoglycemia. Possible causes include an overactive thyroid gland (hyperthyroidism), heart conditions, hormonal disturbances (especially those associated with the menstrual cycle or menopausal, withdrawal from alcohol and drugs, excessive caffeine intake and some psychological disorders. Although blood testing shows that hypoglycemia is not responsible for these symptoms, many people do feel better when they omit sugar from their diet. However, it is still important to search for other possible causes of these hypoglycemic-like symptoms.

Impotence

Another symptom that may occur in the undiagnosed diabetes is impotence. Many men go to their doctor for the first time when this complaint develops. Elevated blood sugars may confirm the diagnosis. With proper treatment, the impotence may disappear. Impotence will be discussed more thoroughly in Chapter 24, "Diabetes and the Man: The Problem of Impotence."

Vascular Disease

Finally, when vascular disease (arteriosclerosis) of the legs or heart (coronary artery disease) occurs at a relatively young age, diabetes may be the cause. This is especially true in women since vascular disease is normally very rare before menopause. Vascular disease is discussed much more thoroughly in Chapter 26, "Complications."

The above signs and symptoms frequently occur when diabetes has not been diagnosed. Early diagnosis can mean early treatment and prevention of some of these serious complications. Prevention is the reason behind many community diabetes awareness campaigns, and are quite effective in educating the general public about these complications. I generally recommend that all people be checked for diabetes, even if they are feeling well, every 6 to 12 months, more so if they have a family history.

5

Making the Diagnosis

Signs and symptoms that should make one suspect diabetes include fatigue, increased thirst, increased urination, change in appetite (often an increase, but sometimes a decrease), weight loss, blurred vision, double vision and other, more subtle, symptoms discussed elsewhere in the book. People can have diabetes and feel perfectly fine, to make the diagnosis one of the following techniques can be used.

Urine Sugar Test

Urine sugar tests are the least reliable of the diagnostic laboratory tests and cannot be used alone to make the diagnosis. Urine sugar tests can be negative despite elevated blood sugar. The reverse can also be true; i.e., urine sugar tests can be positive despite normal blood sugar levels. The following case illustrates this problem.

Years ago, I treated a five-year-old boy who was spilling sugar in his urine. The boy's family doctor had referred him to me because a routine urinalysis indicated the presence of sugar in his urine despite a blood sugar of only 112mg%. The young boy's mother was terribly concerned that her child might have diabetes. Seeing the boy, however, I was impressed by the lack of any symptoms that might indicate diabetes and by a physical examination that suggested excellent health.

Testing his urine for sugar yielded positive results, but a simultaneous blood sugar test result was only 71mg%. Thirty minutes later I repeated the urine test and it still showed sugar. My conclusion (which greatly relieved his mother) was that her boy did not have diabetes but, rather, a low kidney threshold for sugar, causing sugar to appear in the urine even with normal blood sugars. The medical term for this condition is renal glycosuria. It is a benign condition with no increased susceptibility to diabetes. It is because of situations such as this, that urine testing has fallen by the way side for most people concerned with diabetes.

Fasting Blood Sugar Test

A fasting blood sugar is measured when a patient has not eaten or had anything to drink for eight or more hours. In people under the age of 50, normal fasting blood sugar levels range from 50-to-100mg%, depending on the method of chemical analysis. Anything above that range is strongly suggestive of diabetes, although as one gets older (see Chapter 25, "Diabetes After 50"), the fasting blood sugar may get somewhat higher without indicating diabetes. According to the American Diabetes Association, the diagnosis of diabetes is appropriate when two successive fasting blood sugars are over 140mg%. There are world experts who believe this number should be lowered to 125mg%. Note that in the milder forms of diabetes, the fasting blood sugar can be normal or near normal, but blood sugar levels then jump after eating. The following test is useful in these cases.

After Eating (Postprandial) Blood Sugar Test

This test will identify a greater percentage of people with diabetes (especially people with milder forms of diabetes) than the previously discussed fasting blood sugar test. After eating, blood sugar testing can be at one-hour, two-hour, and three-hour intervals following ingestion of food containing 75 grams of carbohydrate. In general, a blood sugar level is considered abnormal if it exceeds 180mg% one hour after eating, if it exceeds 140mg% two hours after eating, or if it exceeds 100mg% three hours after eating. The American Diabetes Association considers two or more two-hour postprandial blood sugars above 200mg% to be diagnostic of diabetes. If the results of these postprandial blood sugars are borderline, the glucose tolerance test may be indicated.

Glucose Tolerance Test

This is by far the most sensitive test for diagnosing diabetes. It is performed early in the morning, after the patient has not eaten anything since 10 PM the preceding evening. A fasting blood sugar is obtained and then the patient is given 75 grams of glucose. Ingestion of the glucose is then followed by half-hour, one-hour, two-hour, and three-hour blood sugar tests. In some cases, four- and five-hour blood sugar tests are also done, especially when early diabetes is suspected. The four- and five-hour blood sugar tests may be abnormally low in early diabetes, as discussed previously. The glucose tolerance tests should be preceded by three days of heavy carbohydrate intake, which makes the test more accurate. Normal results of the glucose tolerance test show the fasting blood sugar below 110mg%, the half-hour and the one-hour level below 160 to 180mg%, the two-hour level below 140mg%, and the three-hour level below 110mg%. The combination of two or more results above these levels, especially if values are well above 200mg% is a strong indication that diabetes may be present. It is important to emphasize, however, that improper food intake, inactivity (such as bed rest when in a hospital) and a number of medications (diuretics, hormone pills, birth control pills, Inderal, and many others) can cause spuriously high blood sugar results. In such circumstances, the glucose tolerance test is not recommended since it could *erroneously* diagnose diabetes. Also, it is not uncommon to see suspiciously abnormal glucose tolerance results return to normal when the test is repeated several weeks later. The explanation for this is not clear, but it illustrates the point that diabetes should not be diagnosed prematurely based on the test results alone. The overall profile of how well the patient is doing is vital to a proper diagnosis.

There is a modification of the glucose tolerance test in

which sugar is given intravenously instead of orally. This test is performed only when patients cannot tolerate taking sugar by mouth because of vomiting.

Steroid Glucose Tolerance Test

The steroid glucose test is sometimes used when the glucose tolerance is normal but there is a history suggestive of diabetes that developed during a period of stress or during pregnancy. This test may help determine whether a patient may be prone to diabetes. In the test, a steroid is given which acts like pregnancy or stress in bringing about glucose intolerance for a brief period following the ingestion of a large amount of carbohydrate. This test is seldom used by the general practicing physician but can be used by research physicians to try to identify those people who are predisposed to diabetes.

6

Home Blood Sugar Monitoring

These days, the fact that patients test their own blood sugar levels has become commonplace. But it took a while for many of today's medical experts to see the value of people with diabetes evaluating their own blood sugar. When home blood sugar tests first became available, some of the most prominent experts scoffed at the idea of patients using these tests on their own. If the sophisticated doctors themselves did not test blood sugars (as they considered it a laboratory procedure conducted most often by a medical technician), how could they allow their patients to do it? What they did not realize was how simple it was (and continues to get). Today, many of those same doctors wonder how anyone with diabetes could get by without blood sugar testing. They reluctantly admit that they were wrong in not recommending blood sugar testing years ago. What a turnaround in their thinking!

These tests are very accurate, and are a great benefit for those patients who experience difficulty in controlling the ups and downs of their sugar levels. The impetus behind the development of these tests was the fact that over 95% of people with diabetes who found it difficult to control their glucose levels at home subsequently achieved good control when they sought in-hospital treatment where blood sugars were done four times per day to help make appropriate changes to get good control. This was true for both Type I insulin-dependent and Type II non-insulin-dependent diabetes. The following illustrates this situation.

For example, Type II non-insulin-dependent people (who take oral anti-diabetes medications rather than insulin) often came into the hospital after experiencing difficulty controlling

28

their disease at home. These patients thought that they needed insulin. However, after being admitted to the hospital, many of them found their blood sugars quickly returning to normal even before their in-hospital insulin treatment was to begin. In the case of the insulin-dependent person with diabetes, it was not uncommon to see rapid improvement in blood sugar levels in the hospital with a considerable reduction in insulin dose. These events prompted the question: If control could be achieved so easily in the hospital, where physical activity is limited, why shouldn't it be as good at home?

The answer was and still is complex. A stressful environment, a hectic schedule, a change in diet, extra nibbling or an unusually active day are all possible explanations for reduced control of diabetes outside the hospital. With the number of factors at play, how could a person with diabetes possibly know what was affecting blood sugar levels?

The advent of home blood sugar tests provided the kind of diagnostic tool that people needed to make such assessments. With these tests, people can monitor the effect that the factors I've just mentioned can have on blood sugar levels, while at home or at the office. For instance, they can see for themselves whether their blood sugar skyrockets as high as their doctor says it will after a hot fudge sundae or even after eating what they would consider good foods such as fruits, juices, crackers and milk. Too much of these foods can raise the blood sugar as much as sweets can. Self monitoring will help the person with diabetes determine the effects of stress from an examination, a job interview, a family confrontation, etc. With this understanding, they can anticipate dips or jumps in their blood sugar before similar circumstances occur in the future and prevent them from happening.

It is not necessary for all people with diabetes to check their blood sugar levels at home. For people with diabetes who have good control of their disease, whose blood sugars are within normal ranges when they visit the doctor, or who have a milder form of glucose intolerance, urine testing may be an adequate, convenient, and inexpensive method of determining whether or not their diabetes is staying in check.

However, for patients with poor diabetes control, particularly
those who cannot correlate their urine test results with their
blood sugar levels for various reasons, blood sugar testing is
certainly preferable.

"Why Blood Sugar Testing is Preferable to Urine Testing"

Blood sugar testing is a much more direct and accurate
reflection of blood glucose levels than is urine testing. As
you'll learn in the following chapter on urine testing, a positive urine glucose test may mean a blood glucose level of anywhere between 100 to 800mg%. This occurs because urine can
be stored in the bladder for up to eight hours before voiding.
Because of this period of urine storage, results of urine testing
may not match results from blood testing.

For instance, blood glucose levels may be 400mg% when
tested four hours prior to voiding, but fall to a more normal
level of 60mg% just before voiding. However, a urine glucose
test done at the time of voiding would be positive for high
sugar despite the normal blood glucose levels. That's because
the bladder would still contain the urine that was formed four
hours before voiding, and this urine would still have lots of
glucose in it, since the blood glucose was then 400mg%. Any
urine that formed as blood glucose levels became normal
would not contain glucose, but would mix with the existing
urine that contained the high levels of glucose. Therefore, the
overall level of glucose in the urine would be fairly high
when tested, even though the blood glucose level had
dropped significantly. This explains the discrepancy between
a urine test high in glucose and a normal blood glucose test.

As discussed in Chapter 7, a "fresh void" or "second
void" might offset the discrepancy somewhat, but there may
still be some variance so that a urine test will not give as accurate a reflection of the blood glucose level as the actual direct
testing of the blood glucose itself. Instances when blood glucose testing is far superior to urine testing is outlined on the
following page:

To Adjust Insulin Dose

Once your doctor gives you the OK, you can adjust your insulin doses based on your blood sugar test results. This is dependent, of course, on whether you fully understand the action of the insulin or insulins you are taking. I'll go into more detail about this in Chapter 9, "Insulin—A Miracle Drug," so be sure to refer to that section for more information.

Pregnancy

With pregnant women, who have diabetes, the goal of treatment is to attain as perfect control of blood sugars as possible. Anywhere between 4 and 7 blood sugar determinations per day may be required so that appropriate adjustments can be made in treatment. Having these tests performed in a clinical laboratory so frequently would be impractical, inconvenient, and irritating. Home blood sugar testing makes it much easier for the expectant mother.

Those Prone To Severe Insulin Reactions

Some people with diabetes have severe insulin reactions that seem to come without warning. Patients who are prone to such sudden onset reactions should find that the discovering of a dropping blood sugar level by home blood sugar monitoring can warn of an impending reaction. This allows them to take steps to prevent this reaction.

Those with High or Low Renal Threshold or with Kidney Disease

Blood sugar testing is also more accurate in patients with kidney disease than is urine testing. That is because a kidney condition can affect the renal threshold, therefore resulting in an unreliable urine test. *Renal threshold* refers to the maximum level of blood glucose that occurs before glucose spills into the urine. If the renal threshold is low (e.g., under 130mg%), a blood glucose test would reflect the normal level whereas a urine sugar test would be high. On the other hand, if someone's renal threshold is high (over 250mg%, for example), the urine glucose test would be negative because it is not as sensitive a test as a blood glucose test, which would indicate a blood glucose level of 230mg% or greater. Also, with a urine test it is impossible to determine specific levels of urine sugar once the sugar starts spilling into the urine; a positive reading could be anywhere from 200 to 800mg%. For all of these reasons, anyone with urinary tract disorders or with unusual renal thresholds should use blood glucose tests. Today, the only reason to use urine testing is when cost is a factor, and possibly for convenience.

Children Under Two

In children under two who are not yet toilet-trained, urine testing can be unreliable and inconvenient. Obtaining the urine specimen is difficult enough, and babies, not having voluntary control of their bladders, just don't give "second voids."

Illness

Insulin-dependent people with diabetes are understandably reluctant to take an insulin dose when ill (especially if unable to keep food down and vomiting) because they fear an insulin reaction. However, omitting an insulin dose can greatly increase the possibility of ketoacidosis. Therefore, it is important to continue with insulin injections, particularly if there is acetone in the urine. Blood sugar tests will show whether or not the blood sugar levels are getting low. In most cases, however, blood sugar levels will not decrease substantially during an illness, even if food intake is less than normal and the usual dose of insulin is taken.

Those Who Suffer a Variety of Symptoms That May Be Confused with Hypoglycemia

As discussed previously, disturbing symptoms that resemble hypoglycemic symptoms can result from various disorders including anxiety, menopause, thyroid problems, heart problems with palpitations, and decreased circulation to the brain. The ability to obtain blood sugars at home the moment the symptoms occur enables the patient to determine whether or not hypoglycemia is the cause of these symptoms.

Perfectionists

By knowing blood sugar levels at any given instant, those who tend toward perfectionism can understand what affects their blood sugar levels and can make adjustments to maintain blood sugar levels as close to normal as possible. In general, it's been found that the more a person tests his blood sugar, the more likely he will achieve good control.

Methods of Determining Blood Sugar Levels

Very easy blood sugar monitoring methods have been devised. A drop of blood and a lab stick are the basic requirements, but a machine may also be used. The drop of blood can be obtained by a finger stick. Don't cringe! There are a number of simple devices currently available that make it

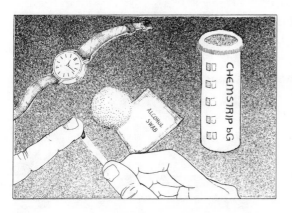

easy to obtain a drop of blood from the finger. Once the blood is drawn, a drop of blood is placed on a lab stick, the results from which can be read by eye or with a machine or meter.

Each procedure used has good and bad points. All strips and/or meters are reasonably accurate if the proper techniques are followed. The strips are inexpensive and disposable. The meters are serviced according to manufacturers' instructions. The choice you make is your own but there are diabetes supply centers, pharmacies, and surgical supply stores throughout the country where you can obtain proper instructions and help to determine the kind of apparatus to use. As an added plus, many medical insurance agencies (Medicare included) have realized the necessity of good diabetes control in warding off medical complications, and are picking up the cost of diabetes supplies. Fortunately, the cost is low to begin with, ranging from 15 to 50 cents, compared to $4-$10 per test in a lab or doctor's office. There are some ways to keep the price of strips down for some people. Discuss this with your physician.

Visual Strips and Meters

Chemstrip bG test strip (Boehringer Mannheim Diagnostics, 9115 Hague Road, Box 50100, Indianapolis, IN 46250; 1-800-858-8072); Glucostix (Ames Division, Miles Laboratories, Inc., Box 70 Elkhart, IN 46515); and the Glucose V test (Caro-Med, Fort Mill, SC 29715; 1-800-328-7397) are several visual strips on the market today. These test kits include a packet of testing strips that indicate results by a change of color. A drop of blood is placed on a strip and after several seconds it is wiped off with a cotton swab. Then colors will appear on the strip to determine analyzes. The colors are compared to those on an eight-block color chart. Using this method, one can

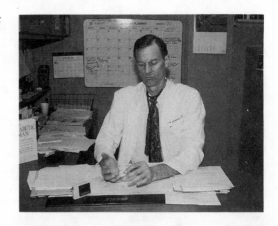

estimate blood sugar levels that range from 20 to 800mg%.

The Accu-Chek Advantage by Boehringer Mannheim Diagnostics; The Precision Q10 and *ExacTech Pen* by Medisense Inc., 1-800-527-3339; Glucometers by Ames Company, One Touch II by Lifescan, Trends Meter by Orange Medical Instruments, 3183 Airway Avenue, Suite F, Costa Mesa, CA 92626; 1-800-527-1151; and Diascan S by Home Diagnostics, Inc., 6 Industrial Way, W., Eatontown, N.J. 07724; 1-800-342-7226 are several meters on the market at this time with more coming soon.

Most meters are simple to use and are not very costly. The cost of strips are the expensive part. Discuss with your doctor or diabetes control center the varying points and what would work best for you.

These are just some of the tests and meters that are currently available. I am sure that there are more to come, each with special points that make one more appealing than an other. Hopefully the competition among manufacturers will bring down the price of the strips. Alternate methods of blood sugar testing—ones that are less invasive—are being developed, such as the one described below.

Man Helped by Home Blood Sugar Monitoring

The following patient exemplifies a case where the advantage of home blood sugar monitoring over urine testing is clear, given this patient's particular circumstances. I began treating this man in 1974, when he started to have bouts of confusion, disorientation, and near blackouts (caused by hypoglycemia) that came on suddenly. These bouts threatened his job as a machine operator. He was stymied by his condition and did not know how to prevent it. Using urine tests to assess his blood sugar control, he did not recognize the cause of his symptoms as hypoglycemia since his urine tests were frequently positive for sugar after one of these spells.

After evaluating his condition, I found that he had prostatism, which meant that he could not empty his bladder completely. I also found that his fasting blood sugar, when tested in the office was frequently under 50mg%, yet at the same time he had high urine sugar levels. I therefore suggested that he lower his insulin dose substantially to avoid his hypoglycemic reactions. He did this for a while, but when he tested his urine and got positive results he became concerned. Thinking that this meant poor diabetes control, he invariably increased his insulin dose. This in turn led to recurrent near-blackout episodes. Finally, blood sugar testing became available to him. After instructing him on its use, he saw the discrepancy between urine sugar and blood sugar tests, as indicated in the following table.

As you can see by the chart, his urine sugar tests were positive when tested before breakfast even though his blood sugar would actually drop to 40mg%. By comparing the two types of tests (urine and blood sugar), it finally became obvious to him that he could not raise his insulin dose based on his urine tests without the possibility of his blood sugars falling below 40mg%. Since he has been testing his own blood sugars, his hypoglycemic reactions have stopped, and his job is still secure! Now, he may even be using one of the simple meters!

	Urine Tests		Blood Sugars (mg%)	
	Before Breakfast	Before Supper	Before Breakfast	Before Supper
July 20	2%	2%	60	100
July 21	1%	trace	85	110
July 22	2%	2%	100	120
July 23	1%	0%	60	40
July 24	1/2%	1/2%	40	80
July 25	1/2%	1%	40	60

Hospital Stay—Another Good Place for Self Blood Sugar Testing

In general, most people rely on doctors and nurses to take over control of their diabetes while they're in the hospital. But, remember: no one can know diabetes as well as the person with diabetes. Also, doctors and nurses can frequently be very busy. To avoid difficulties with control, bring your blood sugar testing apparatus to the hospital. It will assure you that all's going well and may ward off an insulin reaction by alerting hospital personnel that your blood sugar is dropping.

The Meter of the Future: No Blood Sampling Necessary

Recently submitted for approved by the Food and Drug Administration is a new noninvasive glucose sensor called the Diasensor 1000™ manufactured by Biocontrol Technology, Inc (1-412-429-0673). The sensor is devised not to use blood samples, but sends amounts of electromagnetic energy throughout the skin with a probe. Reflected energy is returned to the device, where it is analyzed. It then displays a blood sugar or glucose reading. The device is portable and an unlimited number of readings can be taken thereby lowering the cost of testing. Millions are anxiously awaiting its availability to the public.

See chapter on insulin to see how Home Blood Glucose Testing can be used to adjust insulin.

7

Urine Testing

It has been over 15 years since the first edition of this book came out, and a lot has happened since then in the area of diabetes sugar monitoring—namely that urine testing has been virtually made obsolete by the home blood sugar tests that are now widely available. Many medical experts even question the inclusion of this chapter in the latest editions of my book, asking: "Don't you think urine testing is passe, or outmoded?" I must admit that since I've switched from testing my urine to assessing my blood sugar levels, I've found the latter much more accurate—especially when it comes to fine-tuning the three factors that most affect sugar levels: diet, exercise and medication. So, I've been in favor of home blood sugar testing ever since it became available, especially if expense is not a factor.

You might then wonder why anyone today would use urine testing instead of blood sugar testing. It simply comes down to a matter of expense and convenience (not having to stick one's finger for blood, for example). With most urine tests, a simple trip to the bathroom is all it takes to get the results. By the time voiding is complete, the urine test result is known and the patient has an idea of how well their diabetes control is at the time. Another advantage, as I'll discuss later in this chapter, is that urine testing is still the best way to check for the presence of ketoacidosis.

To better understand how urine tests work, it is important to first understand the concept of the "RENAL THRESHOLD."

The Renal Threshold

The kidneys, which filter the blood of impurities and excrete these impurities in the form of urine, do not allow sugar to spill into the urine until one's blood sugar reaches a certain level. This particular level of blood sugar is called the renal threshold and generally averages between 150mg% and 200mg% (you can ask your doctor to measure your renal threshold). Therefore, if a person with diabetes has a renal threshold of 200mg% and gets a negative urine test, it means his blood sugar has been below the renal threshold for several minutes to several hours.

However, if the same person has a positive urine sugar, it means his blood sugar has been above 200mg% for a certain period of time prior to the time of voiding.

The Meaning of "Second Voided"

A second or freshly voided specimen may better reflect what the actual blood sugar is at the time of voiding. In order to understand this concept, it is important to realize that although urine is formed in the kidneys (as I mentioned earlier, urine is a by-product of blood filtration), it is stored in the bladder for a period ranging from a few minutes to as much as eight hours prior to voiding. Because of the possible duration of urine storage, a *first* voided urine specimen for sugar testing (which consists of urine that has accumulated over a period of time) may not always give as accurate a reading of blood sugar as a subsequent or second voided specimen will, since this is a more recent accumulation of urine.

Thus, to get a better indication of what the actual blood sugar level is at the time of voiding, it is better to discard the first void or stored urine and get a second void or freshly formed urine specimen 30 minutes later (or soon thereafter).

So, for the patient who has an average renal threshold (between 150mg% and 200mg%) and who has no difficulty in completely emptying his bladder, urine testing may give an fair indication of how well the diabetes is being controlled.

Type II non-insulin dependent individuals with diabetes with normal renal thresholds can rely on urine testing to adequately assess sugar control if their urine tests are consistently negative several times a day, and if their blood sugar and glycohemoglobin levels (the index of long-term diabetes control; see Chapter 12, "One of the Latest Tests— Measurement of Glycohemoglobin" for more information) tests are normal during visits to the doctor. In this case, there may be no need for additional home blood sugar monitoring to confirm the results of urine tests.

There are certain situations, however, where urine testing may not be a sensitive enough to monitor diabetes control. For example, people with diabetes with a high renal threshold may obtain negative urine tests at home even though blood sugars are as high as 220-to 300mg% when tested in the doctor's office. Urine testing would also not benefit someone with a low renal threshold. Here the blood sugar may always be in the normal range, but sugar still spills into the urine, a phenomenon that occurs in many people with diabetes. Children and pregnant women often have lower than average renal thresholds. Thus people with diabetes with very high or very low renal thresholds cannot rely on urine testing to guide them in adjusting their diet or education.

Urine testing also falls short when trying to assess how high a positive blood sugar test actually is. It could be anywhere from 200-to 800mg%. Finally, there is the inability to trust the reading of a second void urine test in those who find it difficult to completely empty the bladder during a first void, leaving residual urine in the bladder to mix with the second void urine. This commonly happens in pregnant women, people with a spinal cord disease or injury, those with a neurological disease such as multiple sclerosis, and men with prostate disease. This is a particular problem in people with diabetes neuropathy, when it affects the bladder. In all of these cases, a urine test can be high for sugar, but blood sugar shows normal. In cases such as these, changes in diet or medication cannot be based on urine testing.

When To Test and How To Choose the Best Method

Type II non-insulin dependent people with diabetes can attempt to assess diabetes control by testing their urine before each meal and before going to bed when they first begin urine testing. Any urine-testing method may be used, but Test-Tape is the one most likely to detect sugar in the urine. If all test results are negative for several weeks, then urine sampling should be done after each meal. If tests continue to be uniformly negative, then the test should be performed once per day or twice per week after different meals. Remember: If tests are positive, then it is necessary to test more often and go to blood sugar testing. Illness necessitates more frequent testing, too. People with hypoglycemia or mild diabetes with mild glucose intolerance should also use the above guidelines.

Type I insulin-dependent people with diabetes should test their urine before each meal and again at bedtime. In addition, they should test the second voided specimen. For some people on insulin, especially children with a low renal threshold, the Clinitest two-drop method is preferred. If the test gives the highest reading, it indicates a very high level of sugar and a possible need for more insulin (or less food if the patient has been overeating). This is where a home blood sugar test would be very helpful. So, if you are not already using this method, discuss it with your doctor.

If a person is very prone to changes in blood sugar after eating or after exercise, then he should test with a very sensitive method such as Tes-Tape, Chemstrip, or Diastix before exercising or any other extended activity, such as a long drive, etc. If the tests are negative, he should test his blood sugar and possibly eat more than his usual diet allows, to prevent low blood sugar reactions.

Final Suggestions on Urine Testing

If you are one of the ones who still use urine testing rather than blood sugar tests, record the results of all your tests. If you record your results consistently, you are more likely to notice any pattern that would indicate too much food or too little insulin.

When you write down your test results it motivates you to stay on a diet, especially if you are getting a lot of high test results. Some people think this is a nuisance, especially when they have a good idea what the result is going to be. They know it's going to be high, so they don't test. If they did test, however, and saw the high results, they would be more likely to be careful with their diet, and they would monitor their insulin dosage food intake and level of activity more closely.

Finally, for greater accuracy in determining the degree of diabetes control, you should strongly consider home blood glucose testing which was described in the previous chapter. For those of you who are familiar with blood sugar testing and find it a superior method and its expense no problem, I would still like to emphasize that you **should know how to test urine for ketones or acetone** (as I will describe later in this chapter), just to be sure the dangerous condition of ketoacidosis is not present. Below I'll describe various urine testing products currently available to assess urine sugar and **urine ketone** levels.

Urine Testing Methods for Sugar

There are several methods of urine testing. If you desire to use these instead of blood sugar testing discuss this with your physician.

Urine Ketone or Acetone Testing

Ketoacidosis is a high blood sugar reaction where the kidneys are unable to absorb the extra blood sugar. The glucose spills into the urine, causing removal of water from the blood stream and the body becomes dehydrated. Symptoms of ketoacidosis are increased urination and thirst. During such a reaction, body fats and proteins are sometimes broken down, forming blood glucose, ketoacids, ketones, and acetone.

If high blood sugar levels occur but body fats are not breaking down, there is no acute danger of ketoacidosis. However, when body fats break down and are converted in the liver to ketoacids, the condition becomes more serious. Tests are available to help detect the presence and formation of these ketone bodies. For the well-controlled person with diabetes who is feeling well, there is usually little need to test for urine acetone. But if any of the following conditions occur, urine should be checked for acetone:

- presence of an illness or fever
- urines very high in sugar for three tests in a row on the same day or blood sugars over 300mg%
- symptoms of high sugar, such as dry tongue, thirst, nausea, and excessive urination

The procedures for three common ketone tests are as follows:

- Acetest Tablet (Ames): Place a drop of urine on the tablet. After exactly 30 seconds, compare the tablet with the color chart.
- Ketostix (Ames): Dip the strip in urine. Compare the strip to the chart after exactly 15 seconds.
- Chemstrip K (Bio-Dynamics): Dip the strip in urine, wait 60 seconds, and compare with the color chart.

If ketones are present with high blood sugar, please contact your doctor immediately for advice (see Chapter 10, "Low and High Blood Sugar Reactions: Hypoglycemia and Ketoacidosis" for more information).

8

Oral Hypoglycemic Agents (Diabetes Pills)

People are always hopeful when they get diabetes that they may not need insulin. For many people with Type II diabetes, this may be true. Besides diet, weight loss and exercise, there are oral hypoglycemic agents (so named because they lower blood sugar levels and are taken orally), commonly called "diabetes pills." They were developed with the hope that they would have the same effect as insulin without being injected. They have been used to treat some cases of diabetes since 1956, when the first of these drugs, Orinase (Upjohn) or Tolbutamide, became available. Initially, there was tremendous enthusiasm with their use since they were found to normalize blood glucose levels in 50% or more cases of Type II non-insulin-dependent diabetes.

This enthusiasm was greatly tempered, however, by a research study called the University Group Diabetes Program (UGDP study), which was conducted in 12 centers throughout the United States between 1958 and 1970. In this study, patients were divided into five groups:

Group 1: those on Orinase, 1500 mg/day
Group 2: those on constant dose of insulin
Group 3: those on varied dose of insulin, depending on blood sugar levels
Group 4: those on placebos
Group 5: those on phenformin* or DBI, 100 mg/day

This study caused quite a stir by concluding (and announcing in several United States papers) that the diabetes pill did more harm than good. Because of these results, some

* This drug has since been taken off the market by the FDA because of serious complications that can result from its use.

doctors stopped recommending these pills because of their possible link to heart attacks. However, many other physicians proclaimed the results of the study to be inconclusive and misleading.

One of the major criticisms was that during the course of the study some patients continued using the diabetes pills despite the fact that their blood sugars were not improving and they were not losing weight—two of the prime objectives in the treatment of Type II non-insulin-dependent diabetes. If blood sugars are not improving despite proper diet, a change in medication is indicated. In the UGDP study, however, patients were kept on the same dose of medicine (in the case of Orinase, 1500mg or 3 tablets per day) for *twelve years*! Thus it may have been poor control of diabetes and improper use of medication rather than the adverse effect of the pills themselves, which could have led to the unfavorable results. Each case of diabetes is unique, and proper supervision and adjustment of medication are essential for sufficient control.

Another criticism was that although there were more patients on Orinase who suffered cardiovascular mortality, many of these patients were sicker in the first place. After much investigation, it has been found that the patients treated with Orinase had more cardiovascular risk factors before the study began than those in the other groups. For these and other reasons, the conclusions of the UGDP study were thought to be invalid by professionals. In addition, only to lbutamide (Orinase) and phenformin were studied, so that the findings of UGDP probably should not be considered identical for the other diabetes pills that were not studied; i e, Diabinese, Dymelor, Tolinase, and the ones that just came on the U.S. market in 1984; i.e., Micronase, Diabeta, and Glucotrol, and in 1994 through 1996, Glucophage, Acarbose, and Amaryl. However, the controversial reverberations of the study have had enough of an impact that most doctors believe diabetes pills should not be used by patients who do not commit themselves to a good diet, exercise, and a goal of excellent blood sugars.

How the Pills Work

As indicated in the following table, there were until 1984, four different tablets that were used in the United States: Orinase (Upjohn), Dymelor (Lilly), Diabinese (Pfizer), and Tolinase (Upjohn). These are called first generation sulfonylureas.

Name	Duration of Effect	Typical Dose
First Generation		
Orinase (Tolbutamide)	6-8 hours	250 - 500 mg 1-3 times daily
Dymelor (Acetohexamide)	10-18 hours	250-500 mg twice daily
Diabinese (Chlorpropamide)	up to 24 hours	50-500 mg once a day
Tolinase	up to 12-24 hours	250-750 mg 1-2 times daily

Other drugs that have been used in Europe for over 15 years and have finally been approved in the United States. These may have advantages over the first gerneration sulfonylureas such as greater potency and fewer side effects. These are called second generation sulfonylureas. They include glyburide (Micronase by Upjohn and Diabeta by Hoechst), and glibizide (Glucotrol by Roerig). They are listed in the following table.

Name	Duration of Effect	Typical Dose
Second Generation		
Micronase Glyburide	up to 24 hours	1.25-20 mg daily
Glynase Glyburide	up to 24 hours	1.25-20 mg daily
Diabeta Glyburide	up to 24 hours	1.25-20 mg daily
Glucotrol	up to 24 hours	5-40 mg 1-2 times daily

The latest of the sulfonylurea is glimepiride (Amaryl) by Hoechst. This may be the best, as studies have shown that it decreases the blood sugar with low blood insulin level, suggesting that it lowers blood sugar by helping insulin work at the cell site. The risk of low blood sugar may therefore by less and side effects may be less as well.

Third Generation		
Glimepiride (Amaryl)	up to 24 hours	1-16 mg daily

There are several points to be made regarding diabetes pills:
- The pills are not oral insulin. Insulin cannot be given orally, because it is broken down by the digestive processes before it is absorbed in the bloodstream, where it can take effect.
- These pills can significantly lower blood sugar levels in Type II non-insulin dependent people with diabetes, but only to a small degree in most insulin dependent people with diabetes. Therefore, these pills are most often used in certain cases of less severe, Type II non-insulin-dependent diabetes, generally when the fasting blood sugar is less than 200mg%. Occasionally, in Type II non-insulin-dependent diabetes, especially when the blood sugar is over 200mg%, as occurs in new-onset diabetes, illness, or surgery, insulin may be needed temporarily. Once the blood sugar is back down, the oral medication may then be tried again.
- The exact mechanism by which diabetes pills lower blood sugar is not completely known and may vary from pill to pill. Several of the diabetes pills probably increase the number of functioning receptors, thus allowing insulin to be more effective in lowering high blood sugar.
- Individual oral medications have different durations of effect. This must be taken into account when using different medications.
- Diabetes pills should not be necessarily interchangeable. One drug may simply not be effective in a given patient. In other cases, there may be adverse reactions if one oral agent is substituted for another. Frequently more than two medications can be used.
- Occasionally, diabetes pills can be very long-lasting and cause blood glucose levels to drop dramatically. This effect

is especially apparent when patients are sick and not eating much. Because of this possible effect, I strongly recommend that patients who take diabetes pills should not use them when they are ill unless they know their blood sugar level is high (by testing blood sugars at home).

Who Should Use Diabetes Pills?

I have seen many cases where oral diabetes medications have been particularly effective. Especially in new-onset diabetes where it is not certain whether the patient will be insulin-dependent, these pills may be useful in determining whether or not blood sugars will normalize. Oral agents may also be very helpful for those people whose jobs would be jeopardized if they were placed on insulin. Some companies have established guidelines wherein they will not hire or retain personnel who require insulin for diabetes control. Thank goodness the National Hockey League and baseball leagues haven't adopted such straying policies, or else Bobby Clarke, Catfish Hunter, and many other gifted athletes would have been forced to give up their playing careers unnecessarily. Fortunately, there are many establishments that will hire people with insulin-dependent diabetes, recognizing that these people offer much talent. However, in organizations with less reasonable policies, a job may be at stake. I have seen several people within such organizations do remarkably well in controlling their blood sugars with diabetes pills instead of insulin. These people were highly motivated and knew the importance of exercise and extremely well-controlled diet.

The pills may be helpful in the older person, too, especially if there is a visual disability. If adequate control is possible with the use of these oral agents, diabetes control can certainly be simplified.

Caution

It is critical that people with diabetes who use oral hypo-glycemic agents are aware that there are interactions between these pills and other medications. Large doses of aspirin, Butazolidin (an arthritic drug), and anticoagulants (drugs that prevent clotting of blood) intensify the effects of diabetes pills. Other drugs, such as diuretics (water pills), steroids, nicotinic acid, and birth control pills, may impair the effect of diabetes pills. Because these curious interactions can affect blood sugar control, the use of any drug should be discussed with a doctor.

Also, when diabetes is complicated by kidney, liver, or heart disease, the effect of oral hypoglycemics can be exaggerated. Extreme caution should be exercised in such cases.

There also has been some interest in the use of nutrients in controlling diabetes. The use of chromium (polynicotinate form) up to 200 or 400 mcg has been suggested to lower blood sugar. Vanadium has also generated some interest as a natural product that may lower blood sugar. We are awaiting more data before recommending them unreservedly.

Who Should Not Use Diabetes Pills?

Because many patients balk at the thought of insulin, diabetes pills are often tried with newly diagnosed patients if they can effectively control blood sugars. Only if the pills fail to obtain the desired blood sugar levels (and if other serious medical problems develop) will doctors agree to resort to insulin treatment. There are some cases, however, when these diabetes pills should not be used, especially in light of the UGDP study. The question is: Should these pills be tried out on patients in the first place? The following case illustrates this predicament.

The Lawyer's Case

The case involves a man who is a 45-year-old, overweight (243 pounds) lawyer who had diabetes for about five or six years. Blood sugars were running over 250mg% despite a maximum dose of two different kinds of diabetes pills. His doctor felt the pills were not effective and referred him to the hospital to begin insulin treatment. But lo and behold! Once

Date	Blood Sugar	Diabetes Treatment
April 11	322 — Fasting 273 — 3 PM	Diabinese 500
April 12	292 — Fasting 231 — 3 PM	Diabinese 500
April 13	194 — Fasting 203 — 3 PM	Diabinese 500
April 14	156 — Fasting 142 — 3 PM	Diabinese 250 Dose lowered!
April 15	104 — Fasting 137 — 3 PM	None No pills!
April 16	97 — Fasting 85 — 3 PM	None
April 17	102 — Fasting	None

in the hospital, blood sugars quickly improved as indicated in the following chart.

Why did the blood sugar level return to normal? Obviously, something was done in the hospital that the lawyer was not doing at home. As you have probably guessed, we simply put him on a diet! Stress and strain aggravate diabetes, and in the lawyer's case, this stress led to overconsumption of food. The key question, however, is whether or not the lawyer should have been placed on the pills in the first place. How should blood sugars be controlled at home if the lawyer goes off his diet? In view of the UGDP study, the diabetes pills should probably not have been used in this situation. Diet, exercise, identification of stressors, and an effort to alleviate some of this stress would clearly be the most effective strategy in controlling this lawyer's diabetes, and these methods should probably have been tried in the beginning. Will the lawyer be able to maintain this healthier life-style? Only he can make the decision.

9

Insulin: A Miracle Medicine

Unfortunately, many people with diabetes view insulin injections as some sort of weapon that they should fear. This is a complete misconception. Before insulin became available, diabetes was often fatal. Today, people with diabetes not only survive, but with proper care they can live long, healthy lives. Insulin prevents many diabetes symptoms and contributes to muscle strength and weight gain in thin persons with diabetes. In fact Tim Belknap, Mr. Universe of 1985, has insulin-dependent diabetes. Regarded in this light, insulin treatment should be appreciated rather than feared.

I think it is important to review the history and progress of insulin therapy since this may relieve the anxiety people have about its use. Until the 1980s, insulin was extracted from the pancreas of cows and pigs. In its early form it contained a number of impurities. A large quantity of fluid had to be injected to get a small amount of insulin. Only one type of insulin then existed; i.e., regular insulin, whose maximum effect lasted only six to eight hours, and which had to be given three to four times a day. There were only reusable insulin syringes, and the insulin needles were large and became dull through constant use. The injections were painful and frequent, and caused ugly changes in the skin. The impurities in the insulin caused skin allergies and resistance to the drug's effect. In patients who were resistant to insulin, doses well above 100 or 200 units were sometimes needed to control blood sugar adequately.

Fortunately, much has been done over the years to make insulin easier to use. By modifying regular insulin with varying amounts of protamine and zinc, PZI (protamine zinc insulin) and NPH (neutral protamine hagedorn) insulins were developed in the 1930s and 1940s and were followed by the lente insulins in the 1950s. These new insulins expanded the useful time activity of insulin and allowed many patients reasonable diabetes control with just one or two doses per day.

Insulin became progressively less contaminated by other chemicals due to the tremendous improvement in the purification process. By the 1970s, very purified insulins were available, which markedly reduced allergic skin reactions and prevented the development of large, unsightly indentations at injection sites left by the less pure insulins. In the 1980s, as discussed later in Chapter 30, "Research—Quest For A Cure," human insulins have been added to the purified pork and beef insulins. In addition, the use of these purified and human insulins has been found to be effective in preventing and treating insulin resistance, which was thought to be related to the contaminants found in earlier insulins. As a result, much less insulin may be required in patients who previously needed over 100 units of the less purified insulin.

More purified and concentrated insulin means that much less fluid is needed with each injection to obtain the required dose. If you ever have questions as to which one to use, go for the purest—your physician can help you here. There is no doubt that the insulin of the 1990s is far superior to the insulin of the 1920's. Finally, insulin needles (especially the disposable type) have been so improved that they are now small and as painless as a mosquito bite. In the final analysis, insulin therapy today is much more convenient and much less troublesome than it used to be.

The chart on the following page classifies and describes the various types of insulins that are currently available.

Type of Insulin[a]	Onset of Action[a] (hours)	Greatest Effect[a] (hours)	Duration of Effect[a] (hours)
Rapid acting			
Regular	1/2-1	2-3	6-8
Semilente	1	4-6	8-12
Mixtard[b]			
(Novo-Nordisk)	1-2	2-3	6-8
Novolin 70/30b	1-2	2-3	6-8
Humulin 70/30	1-2	2-3	6-8
Humulin 50/50	1-2	2-3	6-8
Humalog	20 mins.	1-2	4-8
Intermediate Acting			
NPH	1-2	8-12	12-24
Lente	1-2	8-12	12-24
Mixtard[b]			
(Novo-Nordisk)	1-2	8-12	12-24
Novolin 70/30b	1-2	8-12	12-24
Humulin 70/30	1-2	8-12	12-24
Humulin 50/50	1-2	8-12	12-24
Long Acting			
PZI	4-6	14-20	24-30
Ultralente	4-6	14-20	24-30

[a]Although most people tend to respond to the varied insulins as suggested by this chart, there are exceptions. Exercise and site of injection may affect absorption.

[b]Mixtard and Novolin 70/30b are insulins that have a combination of 30% regular insulin and 70% NPH. Because they are premixed, they are especially good for those who have trouble mixing insulin themselves. Humulin 50/50 has 50% Regular and 50% NPH pre-mixed. **NOTE:** Today, all types of regular, semilente, lente, ultralente, and NPH insulins are made by several great insulin-producing companies in varying degrees of purity that go by brand names. Novo-Nordisk makes Novolin human insulin through DNA engineered technique, purified pork, and also a less pure standard insulin. Eli Lilly makes Humulin insulin through their recombinant DNA genetic engineering technique. They also make Iletin II purified pork and/or beef insulins, as well as slightly less purified Iletin I insulins. Most recently Eli Lilly has introduced Lispro or "Humalog" which is the quickest acting of the insulins. It will help prevent the rapid rise in blood sugar after eating. Because it does not last as long as Regular, the chances of low blood sugar or hypoglycemia several hours after eating is less. Novo-Nordisk makes purified pork insulin, Velosulin, NPH, and Mixtard as well as the human regular lente, and NPH Novolin Insulins using their recombinant DNA techniques.

Tips on Insulin Use

The following points highlight the most important information on insulin use.

- Review with your doctor the different insulins available and the type and dose of insulin that is best for you. Recently, it has been shown that better blood sugar control results when insulin is given at least one-half hour before mealtime, especially before breakfast for patients on only one dose. An exception might be in the case where the patient awakens with an insulin reaction; then, part of the meal (breakfast) might be eaten first. Lispro insulin may allow insulin to be given at mealtimes rather than 30 minutes before.
- Some people who need only 1/2 units of insulin may want to use L-40 insulin rather than L-100. Discuss this with your doctor.
- Rotate the site of injection. Any site of injection should not be used more often than once every 15 days. Repeated injection in the same spot may lead to large lumps which, besides being unattractive, may cause variable absorption of insulin and seemingly inexplicable fluctuations in blood sugars.
- Although the site of injection should not be the same each day, it should be understood that the insulin is absorbed

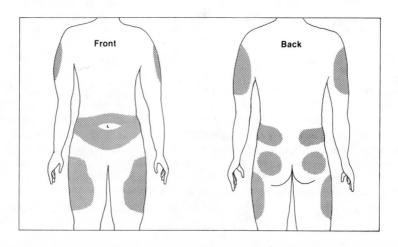

more slowly in the legs than the abdomen, and more slowly in the abdomen than in the arm. Thus, erratic control may result if one day the insulin is given in the leg (resulting in higher blood sugars) and the next day in the arm (resulting in lower blood sugars).

- Since no two people are alike, an identical dose of insulin in two people may have a widely different effect. *That is why it is important for each patient to monitor the effect of the insulin by urine or preferably blood sugar testing.*
- Given the above information, it is advisable to determine how your particular insulin affects you. You should know the onset, the time of maximum effect, and duration of effect. *You can determine how insulin affects you by blood sugar tests 3-6 times per day that will help you determine the proper amount, type, and timing of insulin administration.*

Availability and Storage of Insulin

The following suggestions relate to the availability, storage, and care of the supplies used by insulin-dependent people with diabetes.

- Keep a spare bottle of insulin available to avoid the situation of finding yourself without insulin on a Sunday morning (when most pharmacies are closed) or while on a trip, when insulin may be difficult to obtain.
- A bottle of regular insulin should always be available, even if it is not used daily. It may come in handy, especially during days of illness when blood sugar levels may run somewhat higher.
- Keep the insulin you are using at room temperature. Spare insulin should be refrigerated but not frozen. Present-day insulin will maintain its effect for six months or more at room temperature. Room temperature insulin causes less insulin injection reactions (lumps and bumps) than refrigerated insulin (see the diagram of injection sites).
- Glass syringes may be less expensive than disposable ones, but disposable needles are sharper and less painful. Glass

syringes can be used with disposable needles, thereby cutting back on the expense. It is also possible to use disposable syringes more than once. Discuss this with your doctor.

How To Give Insulin—Single Dose

1. Turn the bottle upside down and roll it between your hands. Never shake it as this will cause bubbles, which can result in faulty measurement.
2. Wipe off the top of the bottle with cotton and alcohol.
3. Pull the syringe plunger to the required number. Put the needle through the top of the bottle and push the plunger down.
4. Pull the plunger to the required number of units of insulin and remove the needle.
5. Wipe the skin with alcohol.
6. Pick up the syringe like a pencil and push the needle straight through the skin. Push the plunger down.
7. Remove the syringe and needle from the skin and wipe the site of injection with alcohol.

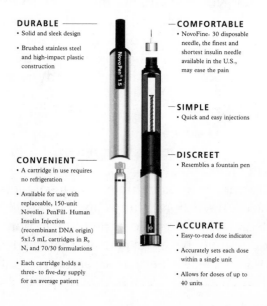

Tip On Insulin Delivery – The NovoPen® 1.5 (The One Dose)

For the convenience of always having insulin available in your pocket or purse, one might consider using the NovoPen® 1.5 or Novolin Prefilled Pen (Novo-Nordisk, 1-800-727-6500) which carry Regular, NPH or the 70/30 pre-mixture in a device shaped like a writing pen. It is very easy to use and has given me very good control. I have enjoyed the convenience of using the NovoPen® 1.5 and its predecessor, NovoPen, for the past 10 years. It allows for added ease and flexibility for those with unpredictable schedules. So, when travelling, or staying late for supper, insulin is always available in a convenient device .

Novolin Prefilled™ Ad from slide

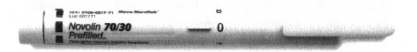

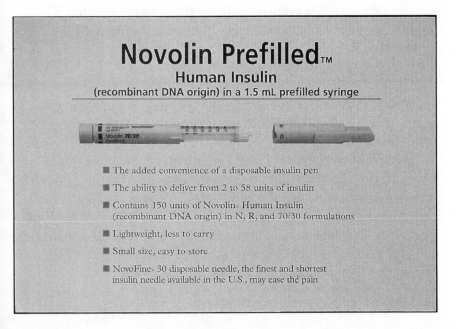

Mixing Insulin

Many use a combination of insulin—Lente and Regular, NPH and Regular, Semilente and Lente, etc.—to achieve good control. When ever using regular insulin with another insulin, however, it is important to avoid introducing any long-acting (NPH or lente) insulin into the regular insulin bottle. Otherwise, erratic control will result. An example of how to mix insulin follows.

If you are on 20 units of Lente and 10 units of Regular insulin in the morning, and 12 units of Lente and 4 units of Regular before supper, you would do the following:

1. Identify both bottles and read the labels.
2. Clean the tops of both bottles.
3. Remove the cap from the needle.
4. Inject 20 units of air into the Lente bottle. Remove the needle from the bottle.
5. Inject 10 units of air into the Regular bottle. Invert the bottle and withdraw 10 units of Regular insulin.
6. Invert the Lente bottle. Carefully insert the needle into the Lente bottle and withdraw the 20 units of Lente. Remember, you already have 10 units of Regular insulin in the syringe, so you must pull the plunger back to the 30 unit mark in order to mix the 20 units of Lente with the 10 units of Regular.
7. Inject the insulin.

For the pre-supper dose, you would follow the same general procedure but substitute the different numbers for the different insulin units.

Comments: If you are using relatively small amounts of Regular or Lispro insulin, the danger of contaminating the intermediate-acting insulin with small amounts of Regular insulin when mixing the insulins is probably insignificant, but care should still be taken. For some people, pre-mixed insulin; e.g., 70/30 may simplify the administration along with the use of the pen devices such as the **Novopen 1.5.**

How To Adjust the Insulin Dose

With experience, many can change their own insulin dose. However, before doing so they should check with their doctors, make sure they are not overeating, and understand the insulin or insulins they are using. To adjust insulin, the guidelines below may be helpful.

Using Urine Tests as a Guide

Before blood sugar testing became available, urine testing had been used to adjust insulin by modification such as suggested below.

Increasing Dose for Those on AM Dose Only
If, while following a proper diet, the second voided urine test before lunch is high for three days or more, Regular or Semilente insulin can be added or increased by 2 units.

If the second voided urine test is very high before supper for three consecutive days, Lente
or NPH can be increased by 2 units.

If the second voided test before breakfast is very high for three consecutive days (and the patient is suffering no insulin reactions during the day), NPH, Lente, PZI, or Ultralente can be increased by 2 units.

Increasing Dose for Those on AM and PM Doses
If, while following a proper diet, the second voided pre-lunch urine test is positive for three consecutive days, the AM Regular or Semilente can be increased by 2 units the next day.

If the pre-supper urine test is positive for three consecutive days, the AM NPH or Lente can be increased by 2 units the next day.

If the bedtime urine is positive for three consecutive days, the Regular or Semilente insulin before supper can be increased by 2 units the next day.

If the pre-breakfast urine is positive for sugar for three consecutive days, the NPH or Lente pre-supper dose can be increased by 2 units the next day.

Adjusting Insulin Using Home
Blood Sugar Monitoring as a Guide

As discussed in Chapter 6, "Home Blood Sugar Monitoring," diabetes is often brought under control very rapidly in the hospital, because of the stable circumstances there. A regular, calculated diet; constant activity so that the body is burning roughly the same number of calories each day; and alleviation from outside stress allows a person to regulate insulin levels. In addition, the doctor makes frequent determinations of blood sugars in order to make appropriate adjustments in insulin dose.

In the past, the doctor discharged the patient once the diabetes was brought under control, only to find that the disease proceeded to go out of control again. Today, however, the patient has the same testing devices available at home as the doctor has in the hospital. So why not monitor your own blood sugars? Once you get the okay from your doctor, you can make some changes in insulin dose based upon blood sugar results. If you are on a regular diet and not overeating, if your activities are relatively constant (for heavy exercise, you may have to eat more food or decrease your insulin dose), and if you understand the insulin or insulins you are using (see chart on insulin actions), you can adjust your own insulin. It should be understood that individual patients need different amounts and different types of insulin. We don't yet know why one 140-pound person may need just 15 units of insulin in one dose of intermediate-acting insulin like NPH, whereas another 140-pound person may need 50 units in two or more doses with a combination of regular and an intermediate insulin to achieve good control. That's why it is important for a person with diabetes to learn with help of Blood Sugar Testing how insulin works on himself.

Increasing Dose for Those on AM Dose Only

If, while following the proper diet, the prelunch blood sugar is over 200mg% for three consecutive days and the other blood sugars are good, 2 units of Regular, or Semilente, or Humalog Lispro insulin can be added, or the Semilente or Regular Insulin can be increased by 2 units (if the person is already on it) to the pre-breakfast longer-acting insulin.

Blood Sugars

Date	7 AM	11 AM	3 PM	9 PM
April 4	80	250*	170	110
April 5	100	240*	150	100
April 6	120	100*	180	150
April 7	90	210*	140	130

Usual Dose: 30 Lente in AM.
*Suggested Change: add 2 Regular or Humalog to 30 Lente in AM.

Comments: The after-breakfast blood sugar is the toughest to keep under control. The body hormones, particularly cortisol, are highest in the morning and antagonize the effect of insulin. Give insulin at least one-half to one hour before breakfast unless Humalog works well to lower the after-breakfast blood sugar.

If the pre-supper blood sugar is over 200mg% for three consecutive days and the fasting and other blood sugars are good, then the pre-breakfast intermediate- or long-acting insulin can be increased by 2-4 units. For example:

Blood Sugars

Date	7 AM	11 AM	3 PM	9 PM
April 4	90	140	210*	150
April 5	120	120	230*	190
April 6	130	150	100*	140
April 7	70	90	280*	160

Usual Dose: 24 Lente in AM.
*Suggested Change: Increase AM Lente to 26 units.

If the fasting blood sugar is consistently over 200mg% and other daytime blood sugars are good, then the intermediate- or long-acting insulin can be increased by 2 units. For example:

Blood Sugars

Date	7 AM	11 AM	3 PM	9 PM
April 4	210*	150	110	90
April 5	240*	130	90	150
April 6	260*	180	70	80
April 7	210*	120	130	120

Usual Dose: 4 Regular, 36 NPH in AM.
*Suggested Change: Make NPH 38 with 4 Regular.

Comments: It is possible that adding more insulin in the morning will result in insulin reactions during the day, which is to be avoided. Eating less supper, or fewer after-supper snacks, may result in lower fasting blood sugars. This might be tried, especially if there is a weight problem. If fasting blood sugars continue to be high, then a night dose of insulin taken either before supper or later at night may be needed to bring the fasting sugar down.

If the 9 PM blood sugar is persistently over 200mg% and other blood sugars are good, then the intermediate- or long-acting insulin can be increased by 2 units. For example:

Blood Sugars

Date	7 AM	11 AM	8 PM	9 PM
April 4	120	140	90	210*
April 5	140	160	90	220*
April 6	90	120	130	240*
April 7	130	90	120	200*

<u>Usual Dose</u>: 4 Regular, 40 NPH in AM.
*<u>Suggested Change</u>: 4 Regular, increase NPH to 42 units.

Comments: Again, there is the possibility that by increasing the AM dose further, insulin reactions or low blood sugars will result before supper. When blood sugars are high after supper, it may be wise to eat less for the evening meal. However, if you are like most of us, you will seldom succeed at this, and so a pre-supper dose of Regular or Semilente may be indicated.

Increasing Dose for Those on AM and PM Doses

If, while following the proper diet, the prelunch blood sugar is over 100mg% for three consecutive days, then AM Semilente or Regular can be increased by 2 units the next day.

Blood Sugars

Date	7 AM	11 AM	3 PM	9 PM
April 4	60	210*	90	120
April 5	70	220*	130	120
April 6	80	250*	100	100
April 7	110	210*	100	80

<u>Usual Dose</u>: 6 Regular, 12 Lente in AM; 4 Regular, 10 Lente pre-supper.
*<u>Suggested Change</u>: 8 Regular, 12 Lente in AM; same pre-supper.

Comments: Again, the blood sugar after breakfast is the toughest to control. The body hormones, particularly cortisol, are highest in the morning and antagonize the effect of insulin. Make sure insulin is given at least one-half to one hour before breakfast.

If the blood sugar before supper is higher than 200mg% for two or three consecutive days, then the AM intermediate-acting insulin can be increased by 2 units. For example:

Blood Sugars

Date	7 AM	11 AM	3 PM	9 PM
April 4	100	140	200*	100
April 5	110	150	270*	70
April 6	130	110	230*	70
April 7	90	90	210*	60

Usual Dose: 4 Regular, 10 Lente in AM; 4 Regular, 8 Monotard in PM.
*Suggested Change: Increase AM Lente to 12 units.

If the blood sugar in late evening is over 200mg% for two or three days, then 2 units of semilente or Regular can be added or increased with intermediate-acting insulin before supper. For example:

Blood Sugars

Date	7 AM	11 AM	3 PM	9 PM
April 4	110	70	150	210*
April 5	60	120	120	270*
April 6	85	120	90	260*
April 7	90	150	80	240*

Usual Dose: 4 Regular,12 Lente before breakfast; 3 Regular, 6 Lente before supper.
*Suggested Change: 5 Regular, 6 Lente before supper.

If the fasting blood sugar is over 200mg% for two to three days, then the intermediate-acting insulin before supper can be increased by 2 units. For example:

Blood Sugars

Date	7 AM	11 AM	3 PM	9 PM
April 4	290*	160	95	75
April 5	280*	150	85	145
April 6	275*	145	125	85
April 7	240*	170	130	130

<u>Usual Dose</u>: 4 Regular,16 Lente before breakfast; 3 Regular, 8 Lente before supper.
*<u>Suggested Change</u>: Increase pre-supper Lente to 10 units.

Comments: It is possible that better control of the fasting blood sugar will result if the Lente is given before bed rather than before supper. Also, there are occasions when insulin reactions or hypoglycemia occur after supper or bedtime. When this happens, the fasting blood sugar may get high because the body produces hormones to counteract the effect of insulin. This has been called the Somogyi Effect (which I will discuss in the Chapter 11: "The Effects of Insulin Over-Use: Brittle Diabetes and the Somoygi Effect") In such cases, the fasting blood sugar may improve with less insulin. Discuss this with your doctor. However, it is probable that improper use of insulin may account for insulin reactions after supper and not enough insulin to keep the AM blood sugar normal.

Increasing Dose for Those on Multiple Doses (MDI) "The Basal—Bolus System"

Many Type I insulin-dependent people with diabetes require insulin by multiple injections or insulin pumps to simulate the release of insulin by the non-diabetic's normal pancreas. This helps them achieve "tight control." By tight control, I mean keeping blood sugars in as close to the 60-120mg% range as possible.

The use of insulin pumps is discussed in Chapter 30, "Research—Quest for a Cure." For those on multiple injections, with pen devices such as the NovoPen® 1.5, or disposable insulin pens, there are various ways to achieve tight control. In general, regular insulin is given in "Boluses" (30-40 minutes before meals). Lispro or Humalog insulin is given at mealtimes to prevent a rise in sugar after eating in combination with long-lasting or intermediate-acting insulin to achieve "Basal" insulin effect. Basal insulin is the insulin needed to prevent the breakdown and conversion of the body's glycogen, fats, and proteins into ketones and sugar and to prevent the diabetes from going out of control. Diabetes can go out of control even when one is not eating, if no basal insulin is present. Ultralente insulin is the preferred long-acting insulin; it is considered relatively "peakless," so that too much of it won't suddenly accumulate in the blood and cause a severe low blood sugar reaction. Because PZI insulin peaks and is known to cause insulin reactions at 2-4 AM, when the user is asleep, it is no longer used to any great extent. Small amounts of Ultralente insulin remain in the bloodstream over a 24-hour period. When intermediate-acting insulin rather than long-acting is given, it is generally given at bedtime as NPH or Lente to give "basal" insulin during the night and to keep the fasting blood sugar normal.

The advantages of this Basal-Bolus System include better control for people with Type I diabetes and less chance of insulin reaction as there is less NPH or Lente to peak at certain times. Without the high doses of NPH or Lente, there is more flexibility so that meals can be delayed without as much risk of hypoglycemia. In addition, with the help of self-blood sugar testing, small changes in pre-meal boluses can be made to allow a little extra in the diet from time to time. To help with this system, a device was introduced in the USA in 1986 by NovoNordisk called NovoPen®. NovoNordisk improved this device by introducing the NovoPen® 1.5. With this device, insulin can be carried with you like your wallet—always there when you need it. This makes your insulin dose available when the proper time comes: for example, before meals.

Finally, there are other devices, called the Medi-Jector (Medi-Ject Corporation, 1-800-328-7074), which deliver insulin by a painless power air spray rather than a needle, thereby lessening the aversion to giving many doses of insulin each day. A young engineer from RCA introduced me to the Medi-Jector (and, as you might suspect, he goes for the best!). It's expensive though; currently, the Medi-Jector retail price is about $595. However, with a doctor's prescription, it may be covered by many insurance plans. This may be especially appealing to parents who administer insulin to their young children.

A particularly gratifying case to me was that of a 16-year-old youngster who was underweight and short in stature. When I first saw him, his blood sugar was over 500mg%. He was concerned about whether anything could be done about his height, just over five feet, and his weight of 99 pounds. I suggested he start using several doses of insulin per day to get better control, but he did not want to take more than one injection a day. This young fellow was a brilliant, all-A student near the top of his high school class, but no matter what logic I used, I could not convince him to take more injections. He did finally agree to try multiple doses with the Medi-Jector, and with improved control he gained 30 pounds and 3 inches in the next year.

In addition to the Medi-Jector, there are two other jet power air sprays that have been made available, the Vitajet (Vitajet Precision Instruments, Inc., 917 Glenneyre, Laguna Beach, CA 92651) and the Preci-jet (Ulster Scientific, Box 902, Highland, NY 12528). My experience with these latter two has been limited, but Barbara Toohey and June Biermann at the Sugarfree Center in Van Nuys, California, report in their Health-O-Gram (Fall/Winter 1985) that experiences of some of Preci-jet and Vitajet users were particularly gratifying.

The following tables show how blood sugar tests might be used to achieve better diabetes control for those taking multiple dose with the Basal-Bolus System.

Increasing Insulin Dose for Those Using Regular in Multiple Doses Plus NPH or Lente

Some people who are aiming for tight control use regular insulin before meals and NPH or Lente at bedtime. This is seen in the following examples with adjustments being made if there is a pattern of high blood sugars at a certain time.

If the 11 AM blood sugars are consistently high, then raise the pre-breakfast fast-acting Regular or Humalog (Lispro) insulin:

Blood Sugars

Date	7AM	11AM	3PM	9PM	2AM
April 5	80	170*	95	75	90
April 6	100	210*	100	80	85
April 7	95	205*	110	120	110
April 8	110	195*	95	85	75

<u>Usual Dose</u>: 8 Regular Humalog pre-breakfast, 8 Regular or Humalog prelunch, 10 Regular or Humalog pre-supper, 16NPH at bed.
*<u>Suggested Change</u>: Raise the pre-breakfast Regular or Humalog to 9 units.

If the 3 PM blood sugars are high, then raise the pre-lunch dose:

Blood Sugars

Date	7AM	11AM	3PM	9PM	2AM
April 5	80	90	190*	98	75
April 6	90	80	200*	68	120
April 7	70	85	195*	89	68
April 8	69	75	220*	68	110

<u>Usual Dose:</u> 10 Regular pre-breakfast, 6 Regular pre-lunch, 9 Regular pre-supper, 20 Lente at bed.
*<u>Suggested Change:</u> Raise pre-lunch to 7 units.

If the pre-bed sugar is consistently high, then raise the pre-supper insulin:

Blood Sugars

DATE	7AM	11 AM	3PM	9PM	2AM
April 5	80	95	90	190*	85
April 6	85	99	98	220*	95
April 7	95	95	78	195*	88
April 8	110	68	78	180*	89

<u>Usual Dose</u>: 9 Regular pre-breakfast, 5 Regular pre-lunch, 8 Regular pre-supper, 20 NPH at bed.
*<u>Suggested Change</u>: Raise pre-supper to 9 units Regular.

If, on the other hand, the pre-breakfast blood sugars are high, then the night NPH will need to be raised:

Blood Sugars

Date	7AM	11 AM	3PM	9PM	2AM
April 5	165*	78	89	99	99
April 6	180*	98	99	100	110
April 7	200*	80	90	120	80
April 8	160*	120	100	85	100

<u>Usual Dose:</u> 10 Regular pre-breakfast, 5 pre-lunch, 8 Regular pre-supper, 22 NPH at bed.
*<u>Suggested Change</u>: Raise night NPH to 23 units.

Comments: Again, it is important to check the 2-4 AM blood sugar to make sure it is not low. If it is low, the Somoygi effect may be taking place, causing a rise in blood sugar in the morning. If it is low, less bedtime NPH may be needed.

I also caution patients about giving extra Regular (as indicated in schedule below*) when an occasional blood sugar gets above 180mg% or 200mg%. If extra Regular is given (1-4 units) the blood sugar may subsequently go low, and a serious insulin reaction can take place. Or even if a serious low blood sugar does not result, sweets or food may be taken to prevent it from going lower, and your weight may go higher than you want.

Finally, all the above changes are based on the assumption that there is no *outside factors*, such as the two most likely culprits: <u>overeating and stress</u>. If it's one of them, that should be worked on first!

*Schedule for Extra Regular Insulin if Occasional Blood Sugar is High (Insulin by Sliding Scale)

Blood Sugar	Extra Regular Insulin
180-239	1 unit
240-300	2 units
300-399	3-4 units
Over 400	Call your doctor if sick or if you have urine ketones

Increasing Insulin Dose for Those on Multiple Doses Using Ultralente

Blood Sugars

Date	7AM	11 AM	3PM	9PM	2-4AM
April 5	90	160*	90	80	80
April 6	100	180*	100	130	110
April 7	90	210*	80	100	100
April 8	90	180*	70	100	80

Usual Dose: 18 Ultralente, 6 Regular pre-breakfast, 5 Regular pre-lunch, 7 Regular pre-supper.
*Suggested Change: Increase 6 Regular pre-breakfast to 7 Regular.

Comments: The above is very close to "tight control." When regular is raised one unit, other blood sugars may start dropping, and insulin may need to be dropped on other scheduled doses.

The 2-4 AM blood sugar has to be watched carefully during this program, as hypoglycemia may occur during this period of fasting, when insulin is not being counteracted as much by the body's hormones because of their low levels at this time of night.

In the same way, if the pre-supper blood sugar is high, the pre-lunch, *not the pre-supper,* insulin should be raised, as seen here:

Blood Sugars

Date	7AM	11 AM	3PM	9PM	2-4AM
April 10	60	110	180*	80	80
April 11	100	80	190*	120	80
April 12	80	105	210*	90	100
April 13	90	80	180*	90	70

<u>Usual Dose:</u> 20 Ultralente, 9 Regular pre-breakfast, 6 Regular pre-lunch, 8 pre-supper.
*<u>Suggested Change:</u> Increase 6 Regular pre-lunch to 7 Regular.

Or, if the bedtime blood sugar is too high, then the presupper insulin may need to be raised, as seen here:

Blood Sugars

Date	7AM	11AM	3PM	9PM	2AM
May 10	80	80	80	160*	80
May 11	100	130	120	220*	100
May 12	90	130	80	220*	120
May 13	120	90	80	190*	130

<u>Usual Dose:</u> 22 Ultralente, 9 Regular pre-breakfast, 6 Regular pre-lunch, 9 Regular pre-supper
*<u>Suggested Change</u>: Raise 9 Regular pre-supper to 10 Regular.

Sliding Scale Insulin

Occasionally, when not sick (<u>when sick,</u> see Chapter 27, "What To Do When Ill" on how to give extra insulin safely), extra insulin may sometimes be given in addition to your usual dose as indicated in the table on the next page .

*Schedule for Extra Regular Insulin. If Occasional Blood Sugar is High (Sliding Scale Insulin).

Blood Sugar	Extra Regular Insulin
180-239	1 unit
240-300	2 units
300-399	3-4 units
Over 400	Call your doctor if sick or if you have urine ketones

Decreasing Dose

Insulin dose can also be decreased under the advice of the physician. In general, if an insulin reaction occurs with an unusual amount of exercise or skipped meals (these are frequently the explanations for unusual insulin reactions, and therefore the insulin dose need not be changed), insulin can be decreased by 2-4 units. The type of insulin decreased will depend on the time that the reactions occur. For instance, if an AM dose only decreases the Regular or Semilente insulin by 2-4 units, then the reaction occurs around noon or before. Decrease the NPH, Lente, Ultralente, or PZI by 2-4 units if the reaction occurs in the late afternoon, evening, or night.

Those who take both AM and PM doses should decrease the appropriate insulin by 2-4 units according to the time the reaction occurs. For instance, if it occurs before noon, Regular or Semilente should be decreased the next day before breakfast. If the reaction occurs after supper but before bed, the Regular or Semilente should be decreased before supper the next day. And finally, if the reaction takes place late at night or before breakfast, the NPH or Lente should be decreased before supper the next day.

Diet and Insulin

Many of the suggested adjustments in insulin dose are needed even when the two critical factors of diet and activity are kept constant. But what happens when diet and activity change? Then, the situation becomes much more tricky. I cannot, for instance, predict exactly what is going to happen when my patients decide to splurge or consume a vastly different number of calories each day. For many patients who suspect that they may deviate from their standard diet on a given day, I try to determine what effect the change in calories will have on their blood sugars, then attempt to make an adjustment in insulin according to the percentage of extra calories they are consuming. It may then be reasonable to take a small percentage of extra insulin to compensate for a heavy meal in order to keep the blood sugar down after a heavy meal.

The drawback to this compensation is that if the number of calories consumed exceeds the number of calories burned by the body, there may be weight gain, especially if the overeating becomes a daily habit. Also, patients should be aware that overeating can accelerate arteriosclerosis. Many diabetes specialists feel that the less insulin that's needed to control blood sugars, the better. Their goal, and I tend to agree with them, is for the patient to eat just enough to maintain good nutrition and strength, so that only a minimum of insulin is needed. Extra calories especially carbohydrates require extra insulin, which thwarts achievement of excellent control with as little insulin as possible.

What To Do When All Blood Sugars Are High

In certain circumstances, blood sugars can rise even if the diet and activity are relatively constant. The hormonal changes involved with pregnancy, menses, and illness can all affect blood sugar control. Since these issues have been discussed in other chapters, I will not discuss them again here. However, there are other times when the blood sugar rises for unexplained reasons. If this occurs, it's important to continue the usual doses of insulin while supplementing them with small amounts of extra regular insulin (see sliding scale below). If blood sugars are high with heavy spillage of urinary acetone, about 20% of the total usual dose of insulin can be given at frequent intervals (see Chapter 10 on ketoacidosis and sick day rules in Chapter 27). When blood sugars are high (over 200-to-250mg%) before meals, without urinary acetone, and the person is not feeling well, about 10% of the usual dose can be given several times a day until blood sugars are back to normal. Then the usual insulin dose should be reinstituted.

It is evident that the advent of insulin has made life healthier for the people with insulin-dependent diabetes, but there are drawbacks if it is misused, or rather over-used, as I will discuss in Chapter 11 on the phenomenon of Brittle Diabetes (diabetes that is difficult to control). Using too much insulin to adjust slight fluctuations in blood sugar levels can actually aggravate the condition in some cases. If you are insulin-dependent, it is vitally important to have a clear understanding of the type or types of insulin you are using, and how their use affects you. This chapter and the following ones should underscore the importance of a good working knowledge of insulin and its use.

Too much insulin also results in hypoglycemia, which is then treated with sugars. Then blood sugar goes back up, resulting in the bouncing blood sugar phenomenon.

Sliding Scale Insulin

To help get blood sugar quickly back to normal, when blood sugars unexpectedly go out of control. Insulin by "sliding scale" can be given. See chart below:

For Blood Sugar	150 - 180	Give 1 Extra Regular or Humalog
For Blood Sugar	181 - 210	Give 2 Extra Regular or Humalog
For Blood Sugar	211 - 240	Give 3 Extra Regular or Humalog
For Blood Sugar	241 - 270	Give 4 Extra Regular or Humalog
For Blood Sugar	271 - 300*	Give 5 Extra Regular or Humalog

*If blood sugar is 300mg% call physician.

Repeat this sliding scale before every meal until blood sugar under 150, then resume usual insulin dose.

Before using the sliding scale consult your physician as to whether it would be appropriate for you.

10

Low and High Blood Sugar Reactions: Hypoglycemia and Ketoacidosis

With diabetes, low blood sugar reaction (or hypoglycemia) and high blood sugar reaction (with ketoacidosis) can be serious conditions. But by understanding how food, exercise, insulin, and diabetes pills affect blood sugar, and how to balance these factors, these reactions can be prevented.

Hypoglycemia

A person usually experiences hypoglycemia when the blood sugar goes below 50mg%. A low blood sugar reaction can be caused by too much insulin, too many diabetes pills, too much exercise, or most commonly, too little food. This last condition usually occurs when a person with diabetes skips some or all of a meal even though he takes his insulin or diabetes pills.

One of the most striking features of a low blood sugar reaction is the speed with which it comes on. A person with diabetes may be feeling fine when, all of a sudden, he gets shaky, nervous, sweaty, irritable and hungry. Sometimes he may cry, become angry, sleepy, confused or complain of blurred vision or headache. If he isn't treated at this point, he may later develop other symptoms such as delirium or increased confusion; he may even lose consciousness or have a seizure.

Any of the above symptoms occurring alone may not pose a danger to most people with low blood sugar and should disappear once blood sugar is back to normal. However, if these reactions occur in certain situations, they can be very dangerous or, if not dangerous, very embarrassing. Driving a car, trying to score two points in an important basketball game, attempting to make a favorable impression on a date or at an important business meeting, may not be a good time to suffer a low blood sugar reaction!!

For the most part, these reactions can be prevented with knowledge of the responses to food, exercise, and whatever insulins or diabetes pills a person may be using. It is also important for him to realize that it takes less than one teaspoon of sugar to go from a normal to a low blood sugar level. Since a fruit exchange or a bread exchange equals two to three teaspoons of sugar, it is easy to see how skipping either exchange may result in a low sugar reaction. Also, exercise causes the body to burn approximately two to five or more teaspoons of sugar per hour. Therefore, if a person with diabetes plans heavy activity or exercise, he should have extra food available, preferably the quick-acting kind, like sugar tablets, soda, orange juice, or sherbet. He should be able to judge the amount of sugar contained in a given portion of food and to compensate for any anticipated exercise.

He will easily be able to learn how much he needs by trial and error. Blood sugar testing will be very helpful in this regard, though some people still use urine testing. If urine is negative for sugar before exercise or the blood sugar is below 100mg%, eat at least the amount of food equal to two to five teaspoons of sugar before rigorous exercise and maybe every half-hour to hour afterward.

As previously mentioned, know as much as possible about the insulins or diabetes pills you are using. Most often, Regular or Semilente insulins have their greatest effect within four hours; NPH and Lente have their greatest effect within 10 hours; and Ultralente and PZI have their greatest effect 16 hours later. At these times of greatest insulin effect, low blood sugar is most likely, but a low sugar reaction can occur at any time, especially if a meal or part of a meal is skipped. Diabetes pills such as Diabinese, Dymelor, Tolinase, Micronase, Diabeta, Glucotrol, Orinase and Amaryl can also lower the blood sugar significantly. Thus, anyone taking any of these pills should be especially careful not to skip meals, especially with exercise.

Finally, if a low sugar reaction does occur, sugar is needed immediately. If conscious, he can take four ounces of orange juice or soda, two lumps of sugar, two teaspoons of cola syrup, or seven to eight Life-Savers or Charms. Better and faster acting are glucose tablets, of which he can take three or four. Currently available are *Dex 4 or B-D Glucose Tabs* . If these sugar sources do not alleviate the low sugar symptoms within a few minutes, ingestion of the same amount of sugar can be repeated. If the person with diabetes is not cooperative or is unconscious, he can be given a concentrated sugar by mouth, such as Instant Glucose, Reactose Paste, or a "Cake Mate" (a decorative icing found in supermarkets). This must be done carefully. Even though unconscious, a person should be able to swallow just as he does when he is sleeping. Put small amounts in the mouth. Within minutes, there should be improvement.

If none of these alternatives work quickly, glucagon, an injection that raises blood sugar, should be administered by a friend, family member, doctor, or anyone else who is present and understands the procedure.

Like insulin, glucagon is a hormone produced in the pancreas. Whereas insulin is produced in the beta cells in t he pancreas, glucagon is produced in the alpha cells (which are adjacent to the beta cells). While insulin *lowers* blood sugar, glucagon raises blood sugar. Like insulin, glucagon can be extracted from the pancreas in a powder form, available to treat severe insulin reactions. It can be administered as follows:

1. Diluting fluid is available in a syringe (Eli Lilly).
2. Inject all the fluid into the bottle with the glucagon powder in it.
3. To mix, rotate bottle in hands. When mixed, it will look like "sugar water."
4. Withdraw one-fourth to one full syringe of the mixture (the exact amount is not as critical as it is in the case of insulin).
5. Select an injection site in the upper arm.
6. Inject the entire amount in the syringe just as you would with insulin.

Within 5 to 10 minutes, the person should awake and be able to eat. Glucagon raises the blood sugar quickly, but does not maintain it for more than a short period. Once the person with diabetes responds to the glucagon, he should be given food, preferably simple sugar. In all such severe cases, the doctor should be notified immediately or the person with diabetes should be brought to the hospital, unless those who administer the glucagon are very familiar with treating such insulin reactions.

After such a severe reaction, a person generally feels "washed out," with a headache and nausea for several hours, but suffers no serious consequences. It should again be emphasized that there is usually an explanation for such severe reactions: omission of food, extra activity not compensated for by extra food, or improper insulin dose. With proper attention and care, these reactions should be avoidable.

The Doctor Suffers Hypoglycemia

Like many people with diabetes, I too suffer hypoglycemic spells from time to time. One of these episodes occurred one night after a long day's work and a rigorous tennis match. I had apparently underestimated the number of calories I had burned that day and woke up at 2 or 3 AM in a sweat, feeling somewhat weak. Not feeling quite awake, I woke Maureen from what had been a peaceful night's sleep to request that she get me something to alleviate my low blood sugar. Half awake herself, she replied, "What do you want, some orange juice? More awake by now, I replied, "No, but can you make me a roast beef sandwich?" Maureen's predictable response to that request was, "If you're alert enough to want a roast beef sandwich, you can go make it yourself!" Too tired for that, I settled for some orange juice.

Ketoacidosis

The other reaction of concern is a high blood sugar reaction with acidosis, called diabetes ketoacidosis. This condition is extremely serious since, once it occurs, it is estimated that 5-10% of patients can die, especially if good medical care is not readily available. It must be emphasized, however, that this condition is avoidable under almost all circumstances.

I have seen patients who have been hospitalized 4 or 5 times per year with ketoacidosis. One patient was hospitalized 20 times in one year. After coming under my care, he finally learned how to prevent it, and no subsequent hospitalization was needed. I would like to think of myself as the hero who helped this man overcome the problem that nobody else could, but all I did was give him some basic information (far from a heroic task) and motivate him to be more attentive to his diabetes. Some of this basic information follows.

First of all, this condition results from insulin deficiency. Most Type II non-insulin-dependent people with diabetes don't have to worry about ketoacidosis since they usually have high levels of blood insulin. However, some patients who were initially diagnosed as being Type II non-insulin-dependent may eventually develop Type I insulin-dependent diabetes, especially if a serious illness occurs. Therefore, it is important for both Type II non-insulin-dependent and Type I insulin-dependent people with diabetes to be aware of the basic facts concerning ketoacidosis.

When insulin deficiency occurs, a chain of events follows. Without insulin, the blood sugar cannot be escorted across cell membranes, nor can it be utilized or stored properly. Thus, blood sugar goes up. Elevation in blood sugar is accentuated by a process called *gluconeogenesis*, which means new formation of glucose. This process occurs in the liver when insulin is deficient. During gluconeogenesis, glucose is formed from certain amino acids and glycerol. This point is very important since it explains why the blood sugar can get high even when the person with diabetes is not eating any food or sugar. It is also the reason why Type I people should probably not omit an insulin dose even if there is nausea or vomiting.

As the blood sugar gets higher, the kidney is unable to absorb all the glucose and thus glucose spills into the urine. High glucose levels in the urine result in removal of water from the bloodstream. Increased urination occurs, and the body becomes dehydrated, thus causing increased thirst. If caloric fluids such as orange juice (even the unsweetened kind) or milk are consumed to quench the thirst, the condition can become even worse, causing further elevation of blood sugar and further urination, so that thirst and dehydration become even greater.

Other symptoms associated with insulin deficiency and/or high blood sugar include blurred vision, muscle weakness, fatigue, lethargy, irritability, and interrupted sleep associated with excessive urination. Through the kidney, there is also loss of body minerals, such as sodium, potassium, phosphorus, and possibly calcium.

The above discussion explains the blood sugar elevation and some of the symptoms of insulin deficiency, but these conditions can all be present without acidosis. Over a prolonged period of time, high blood sugar may add to the chronic complications of diabetes but there is no acute danger.

It is only when high blood sugar is associated with acidosis that a very threatening condition arises. People with diabetes become prone to acidosis when a more severe insulin deficiency occurs in combination with excessive production of glucagon. Fatty tissue then releases fatty acids which, by themselves, may not be dangerous. However, when these fatty acids are converted in the liver to acid bodies, called acetoacetate and beta-hydroxybutyrate, they become dangerous since excess acids cause the blood pH to drop below the normal range of 7.35-7.44. The resulting acidosis, along with high blood sugar, dehydration, and mineral deficiency, affects cellular function. If this condition is severe enough, it can lead to death.

Because of the seriousness of this condition, it is important to understand why it occurs and to prevent it from happening. In my experience, it is most likely to occur in the following circumstances:

◆ In the person who omits his insulin dose.
◆ In the person with new-onset diabetes who is not aware that his body lacks insulin.

- In the Type I insulin-dependent person who overeats or overdrinks, especially highly caloric drinks such as milk, juice, or soda, so that he becomes relatively insulin-deficient even though he is taking insulin. In the insulin-dependent person with diabetes who is ill. Even a minor illness can apparently increase the demand for insulin so that more is needed to overcome the insulin resistance that develops with an illness.

- Under severe emotional stress. This is particularly common in teenagers, when puberty and the struggle for self-sufficiency can cause hormonal changes that can make them relatively insulin-deficient and therefore more susceptible to ketoacidosis.

- Although I have not actually seen this, it is reported that heavy exercise in patients with poorly controlled diabetes can actually aggravate the diabetes state rather than improve it.

Knowing that acidosis is more likely to occur in the above circumstances, the next step to prevention is to be on the lookout for signs that diabetes may be getting out of control. Unlike a low blood sugar reaction, which can occur very rapidly, there are many signs and symptoms that last hours, days, and even weeks to forewarn the person with diabetes of ketoacidosis. As discussed, these symptoms include increased urination, thirst, fatigue, lethargy, blurred vision, and irritability. As the condition progresses, the urine tests become high in sugar and acetone (or ketones) and nausea, vomiting, and weight loss ensue. Finally, deep breathing (called Kussmaul breathing), dry tongue and mouth (indicating dehydration), and progressive mental symptoms, possibly leading to unconsciousness, indicate that acidosis may already be present in varying degrees and immediate contact with a physician is advisable.

The next step toward prevention of ketoacidosis is to give more frequent doses of insulin whenever early signs of uncontrolled diabetes are combined with high urine sugar (or high blood sugars) and urine acetone. This is a crucial step.

When treating ketoacidosis in the hospital, doctors have found that the amount of insulin required is far less than we used to think necessary to treat the condition. Doctors now treat ketoacidosis with relatively small doses of insulin but the doses are *frequently* given (with very high success). The important point is that, if it takes far less insulin than we used to think to treat the ketoacidosis once it has occurred, then it should take even less extra insulin to prevent it from happening in the first place.

In my experience, frequent small doses of extra regular insulin can be given if there is high urine sugar associated with high blood sugar or urine acetone. There are many people with diabetes who are extremely sensitive to regular insulin when their control of the diabetes is good, so that they may have a severe insulin reaction with regular insulin. However, when their diabetes is out of control and acetone or ketones are present in the urine, there is "insulin resistance," so that extra regular insulin is vital to overcome the poorly controlled diabetes. In general, the amount of extra regular insulin that can be given (at a frequency of every two to four hours) is 20% of the usual daily dose as long as the urine stays high for sugar and acetone. For example:

Person A, whose usual total insulin dose is 20 units per day, would give an extra 4 units Regular (20% or 1/5 of 20) every two to four hours until the urine sugar goes under 1% or the blood sugar goes under 180 mg%, as shown in the following table.

Time	Blood Sugar	Urine Sugar	Urine Acetone	Extra Regular Needed	Usual Insulin Dose
7 AM	Over 240	2%	high	4 units	4 Regular, 8 Lente at 7 AM
10 AM	Over 240	2%	high	4 units	
12 noon	Over 240	1%	high	4 units	4 Regular, 4 Lente at 6 PM
3 PM	less than 180	1/4%	moderate	none	

Time	Blood Sugar	Urine Sugar	Urine Acetone Needed	Extra Regular	Usual Insulin Dose
6AM	Over 240	2%	high	12 units	10 Regular, 20 Lente, AM
8AM	Over 240	2%	high	12 units	
10 AM	Over 240	2%	high	12 units	10 Regular, 20 Lente, PM
12 noon	Less than 180	0%	moderate	none	

Person B, whose usual total insulin dose is 60 units per day, would give 12 extra Regular (20% or 1/5 of 60) every two to four hours until the urine sugar goes under 1% or blood sugar goes under 180 mg %, as shown in the following table or some people can give extra insulin according to the sliding scale technique below.

Blood Sugar	Extra Regular Insulin
150-180	1 unit
181-210	2 units
211-240	3 units
241-270	4 units
271-300	5 units

When taking extra insulin, the following points are important:

◆ For those using urine tests, if there is any concern about giving extra insulin for fear it may cause an insulin reaction, home blood sugar monitoring is a helpful guide. If blood sugars are above 240 mg%, the extra insulin is probably needed.

◆ The patient should continue to take the usual doses of insulin along with the extra insulin.

◆ The high urine acetone may persist for several hours after the blood and urine sugars go down since it takes several hours for the body to get rid of the extra acetone. As long as the urine and blood sugars are good, there is no cause for alarm even if the acetone does persist for several hours.

◆ Generally, vomiting from a viral illness does not last longer than four hours. If vomiting should persist more than four hours, a physician should be contacted.

	Too Low	**Too High**
Cause	Too much insulin or exercise and not enough food	Omission of insulin dose or too little insulin; infection, illness, stress
Preceding Warning	Peculiar behavior, or sudden onset in healthy person, or no warning	Tiredness, thirst, frequent urination, fever; illness frequently present
Onset	After short period of peculiar behavior or possibly no warning, sudden loss of consciousness, and convulsions	Several hours to days of above symptoms leading to greater drowsiness and eventual unconsciousness
Appearance	Looks like person is sleeping; sometimes there is muscle twitching and sweating	Person looks very sick; has dry coated tongue; sometimes skin is red and dry
Breathing Pattern	Normal	Heavy, deep
Urine Sugar	Usually negative with no acetone	High sugar and acetone results
Response to Glucose or Glucagon	Rapid – within minutes	None
What To Do	Give sugar or glucagon and call physician immediately	Give insulin and call

For further information, see Chapter 27, "What To Do When Ill." A diet similar to the one in that chapter should be followed until the blood sugars are well controlled.

A summary chart on the preceding page highlights the major differences between low and high blood sugar levels follows.

Importance of Identification

Because high or low blood sugar levels can cause abnormal mental symptoms or unconsciousness, the person with diabetes should wear some form of identification. This identification should give the person's name, address, phone number, doctor's name, and type and dose of insulin or other medication so that proper care can be provided in an emergency. Identification forms, bracelets, etc., available from the American Diabetes Association, the Medic Alert Foundation, and some of the pharmaceutical firms, and are especially useful for those people with diabetes who are prone to insulin reactions.

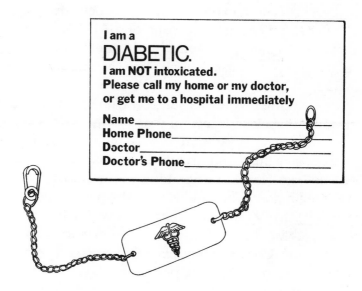

11

The Effects of Insulin Overuse: Brittle Diabetes and the Somoygi Effect

Insulin is by far the most important discovery in the field of diabetes management for the Type I or insulin-dependent person with diabetes. This medication, combined with a proper diet and physical activity, can allow a good, healthy life for many of those with diabetes. However, it is important for the patient who needs insulin for blood sugar control to understand how the various types of insulin work. Without this understanding, there can be needless difficulties with control, and it is not uncommon for these patients to develop what is erroneously described as "brittle diabetes" (a condition where blood sugar levels inexplicably fluctuate between low and high after slight changes in insulin dose, diet or physical activity). In fact, the symptoms result, not from brittle diabetes, but from the misuse of insulin. The following cases illustrate my point.

The first case involved a surgeon who had had insulin-dependent diabetes for several years. In the mornings, he would often experience symptoms of high blood sugar, along with excessive thirst and urination. In an attempt to decrease his blood sugar levels, he would continually increase his usual insulin dose. The trouble was, the type of insulin he was using was PZI insulin, which, you will notice from the following chart, does not begin to take effect until six hours after injection. Consequently, his blood sugars would not come down during the early part of the day; sometimes his levels would get as high as over 400mg%. These symptoms greatly disrupted his operating room schedule. So, he would continue to increase his PZI dose to over 60 units, until the insulin would finally take effect late in the afternoon or early evening. During these times he would often suffer from a severe insulin reaction, where his blood sugar level would plunge drastically.

As I mentioned in the chapter on insulin, there are a variety of insulins, all with specific times of onset and lengths of activity. The following chart shows you the various types of insulin available. It is vitally important to match a patient, with his or her individual blood sugar needs, to the right kind of insulin.

Type of Insulins	Onset of Action[a] (hours)	Greatest Effect[a] (hours)	Duration of Effect[a] (hours)
Rapid acting			
Humalog	20 minutes	1/2-2	4-8
		30 min - 2 hrs	
Regular	1/2-1	2-3	6-8
Semilente	1	4-6	8-12
Novolin 70/30[b]	1-2	2-3	6-8
Humulin 70/30	1-2	2-3	6-8
Humulin 50/50	1-2	2-3	6-8
Intermediate Acting			
NPH	1-4	8-12	12 24
Lente	1-4	8-12	12 24
Novolin 70/30[b]	1-2	8-12	12 24
Humulin 70/30	1-2	8-12	12 24
Humulin 50/50	1-2	8-12	12 24
Long Acting			
PZI	4-6	14-20	24-30
Ultralente	4-6	14-20	24-30

[a]Although most people tend to respond to the varied insulins as suggested by this chart, there are exceptions. Exercise and site of injection may affect absorption site.
[b]Novolin 70/30[b] are insulins that have a combination of 30% regular insulin and 70% NPH. Because they are premixed, they are especially good for those who have trouble mixing insulin themselves. Humulin 50/50 has 50% Regular and 60% NPH pre-mixed.
NOTE: Today, all the types of Regular, Humalog, Semilente, Lente, Ultralente, and NPH insulins are made by several great insulin-producing companies, in varying degrees of purity that go by brand names. Novo Nordisk makes Novolin human insulin, purified pork, and also a less pure standard insulin. Eli Lilly makes Humulin insulin through their recombinant DNA genetic engineering technique. They also make Iletin II purified

pork and/or beef insulins, as well as slightly less purified Iletin I insulins. Novo Nordisk makes purified pork insulin, Velosulin, NPH, and 70/30 as well as the Human Regular, Lente, and NPH 70/30 Insulins using their recombinant DNA technique.

I, therefore, suggested that he take a combination of Regular and Lente insulins one-half hour before breakfast (so that it would take effect more rapidly), plus a small dose of Lente in the evening to keep his sugars down in the late evening and early morning. As the chart shows you, Regular insulin begins acting one-half to an hour after injection and its duration of effect is between 6-to-8 hours. Lente insulin begins acting 1-to-2 hours after injection, and its effects last between 12-to-24 hours. As a result, the surgeon's blood sugar level was rapidly controlled with about 30 percent less insulin than he had been taking. In other words, he got better control with less insulin. Thereafter, problems in the operating room were alleviated, and his severe insulin reactions disappeared. A case of "brittle" diabetes was cured.

This case indicates that poor control of diabetes can often be alleviated simply by understanding how the various types of insulin work. The surgeon simply did not know about the onset, activity, and duration of the type of insulin he was using, because he had not been instructed on the particular characteristics of the various insulins. I have seen countless cases similar to this one where patients did not know the basics of insulin therapy. Once they were enlightened, however, they did fine! The following cases also illustrate obvious over-use of insulin.

Other Cases of So called "Brittle Diabetes" Caused by Too Much Insulin

Some patients show obvious signs of having taken too much insulin. The two following cases of mine are classic examples.

A 22-year-old woman, whom we will call "Jane," with a history of diabetes of 12 years, duration sought my attention for uncontrolled diabetes. She continually experienced very low, followed by very high, blood sugars. Her severe insulin reactions were typically followed by blood sugars in excess of 300-to-400mg%. Upon my evaluation, I found that she had been taking over 100 units of insulin a day, involving a combination of 68 units of NPH and Regular in the morning and another combination of 48 units of NPH and Regular insulin in the evening. In addition, Jane was considerably overweight. Her weight problem was the clue that told me that Jane was getting too much insulin.

What was happening was that her blood sugars would get low every morning between 10 AM and noon. She would then consume large amounts of sugar and other foods (low blood sugars create voracious appetites), and as a consequence, her blood sugars would bounce back up. By the time she contacted her physician in the afternoon, her blood sugars would already be in the 300-400mg% range Her physician would continually increase her insulin dose, fearing that Jane would develop ketoacidosis (a high blood sugar reaction; this problem will be described in detail in Chapter 10, "Low and High Blood Sugar Reactions: Hypoglycemia and Ketoacidosis") and uncontrollable diabetes. However, the increased doses of insulin only aggravated the problem.

I, therefore, decided to cut her insulin dose to approximately 40 units a day, with small doses of Regular and NPH both in the morning and evening. Again, if you refer to the insulin activity chart, you will find that Regular insulin begins acting 1-to-2 hours after injection and its effects last up to 8 hours; NPH insulin also begins acting within 1-to-2 hours after injection and its effects last up to 24 hours. Soon thereafter, Jane's severe hypoglycemia and the "brittleness," or uncontrollable nature, of her diabetes was soon alleviated. As an added plus, she found her weight falling to a much more desirable level.

The third case involves a patient who was at the other end of the age spectrum. Seventy-year-old Viola had been in and out of the hospital on a monthly basis because of high and low blood sugar reactions. Her family brought her to me for an evaluation because Viola was getting increasingly confused and lethargic, and was described as becoming senile and forgetful, not remembering such important things as whether or not she had taken her insulin.

During my evaluation, I found that Viola, who was only slightly over her normal expected weight, had been taking 60-80 units of insulin a day in varied combinations, plus Regular insulin on a "sliding scale" whenever her blood sugars were high. Despite this very high dose of insulin, the degree of her diabetes control, as reflected by her high glycosylated hemoglobin or hemoglobin A1C counts (15.2%), was very poor.

After I modified her diet, insulin and blood sugar testing, Viola improved remarkably. I adjusted her insulin dose from more than 70 units a day to 22 units (16 units of Novolin 70/30 in the morning and 6 units of the same again at night). Her severe hypoglycemia episodes disappeared during the ensuing 8-to-10 months, and her glycosylated hemoglobin count fell to 4.8% during that time as well, despite the tremendous cutback in her insulin dose. As her severe hypoglycemic reactions disappeared, so did her symptoms of senility.

Not-So-Clear Cases

As I've mentioned, the three above cases are clear examples of poor diabetes control brought on by taking too much insulin. In contrast, there are cases that do not so clearly point to an over-use of insulin where episodes are more subtle and difficult to identify. These cases, like the more obvious ones, are also triggered by too much insulin, but unlike the others are followed by an undetectable hypoglycemic episode after which, seemingly without reason, the blood sugar becomes elevated. Once the patient senses that blood sugars have become high, and not realizing that the body is responding to a slight hypoglycemic episode, he or she may incorrectly increase insulin doses. This only serves to renew the cycle of low followed by high blood sugars, aggravating rather than treating the condition.

It has been observed that many people with diabetes with

this problem frequently wake up in the early morning with high blood sugars, unaware that their levels had been low during the night. These patients may have an accompanying headache or morning nausea. They then incorrectly increase their insulin dose.

What I thought to be happening in this type of more subtle episode is that when the blood sugars become low in response to excessive insulin, the body's "counter-regulatory hormones," which include adrenaline, cortisol and possibly growth hormone, come into play. These hormones counteract the sugar-decreasing effects of insulin by pushing the blood sugars back up to high levels even though the person has not been eating. Consequently, a vicious cycle can ensue if the insulin dose continues to be raised in an attempt to prevent subsequent fasting high blood sugars.

Therefore, a vital step to avoiding the drastic fluctuations in blood sugar levels that could develop into brittle diabetes is to be aware of the physiological changes that lead to the problem. These changes were first described by diabetes researcher Michael Somoygi, Ph.D. in 1938, and thus named the "Somoygi Effect." His initial report about the effect appeared in the proceedings of The Society of Experimental and Biological Medicine (Vol:38,1938). But it was not until a second report published in the late fifties (American Journal of Medicine; Vol:26,1959) that it finally became well accepted among practitioners treating diabetes.

The Somoygi Effect: A Cause of Brittle Diabetes?

Excess insulin was thought to cause the Somoygi Effect, a rise in blood sugar levels that can occur with insulin overuse. This can lead to brittle diabetes, where diabetes becomes exacerbated and difficult to control. The problem is that many people don't realize they have taken excess insulin. Essentially what happens is that when too much insulin is taken, hypoglycemia results. This low blood sugar triggers a series of physiological responses that counteract the insulin effect, and blood sugars then bounce back up as the insulin effect is "waning". Thus, there is a tendency for blood sugars to vacillate between low and high without the obvious trigger mechanisms of too much or too little food or exercise.

If patients could recognize the Somoygi Effect, some cases of brittle diabetes would be eliminated. It is important to see if hypoglycemia is preceding the episodes of high blood sugar. This can be done by testing the blood sugar frequently.

Identifying the Somoygi Effect

To diagnose the Somoygi Effect, episodes of hypoglycemia must first be identified. To do this, frequent blood-sugar testing needs to be done. And this frequent testing should be done throughout the day—particularly during the early morning hours between one and four AM. If hypoglycemia is identified, the proper adjustments in insulin can be made to avoid both the hypoglycemic and high blood sugar that follows.

It is essential to consider the possibility of the Somoygi Effect whenever someone with diabetes has unexplained high blood sugars (that is, high blood sugars that do not result from too much or too little food or exercise) or has brittle diabetes—diabetes that is consistently difficult to control. It is also important to consider the overuse of insulin anytime blood sugars are bouncing from low to high after a very large dose of insulin, such as that evidenced by the first three cases discussed above.

It is the experience of many diabetes specialists that better diabetes control can result from a much smaller amount of insulin than many people use. If you think the Somoygi Effect or the over-use of insulin could be a problem, discuss this possibility with your doctor to get the right type and dose of insulin as well as review your diet and exercise prescription.

Other Cases of Brittle Diabetes and Help in Their Management

There are some people with diabetes who are exquisitely sensitive to small changes in insulin, diet, activity or stress.

These patients have true brittle diabetes. So minimal are the changes that patients can't discern any logical explanation for their blood sugars being high one moment and low the next. These patients, when evaluated by their diabetes specialist, frequently show no obvious medical complications to explain their erratic diabetes (for example, diabetes neuropathy, a disease of the nervous system that may occur with diabetes of long duration; it can cause brittle diabetes by interfering with stomach emptying and can affect the counter regulatory hormones such as glucagon, adrenaline and others), leaving their doctors baffled. Here are the stories of two of my patients who had extra-sensitive diabetes.

Calories, Carbohydrates and Diabetes Control

The first patient was 60-year-old Mary Rose Smith, who had had diabetes for over 25 years. She was utterly frustrated with the inability to adequately control her diabetes. She had gone from doctor to doctor, including many diabetes specialists—even seeking treatment at a university medical center and trying an insulin pump, a portable infusion device that delivers a steady amount of regular insulin throughout the day.

When she finally sought my attention, I found her physical examination striking. Despite her 60 years, she was a good-looking woman. She had no evidence of age-related or diabetes-related problems, such as heart, kidney or nerve disease. She did mention having a history of many insulin reactions, which were followed by high blood sugar, and said that she felt equally miserable when her blood sugar level was at 40mg% or 400mg%. I eliminated a possible Somoygi Effect by first cutting back on her insulin and allowing her sugars to run high, then again adjusting the dose to avoid hypoglycemia and the associated rebound phenomena I discussed earlier.

For her part, Mary Rose was very diligent in her efforts to control her diabetes, consuming 1300-to-1500 calories a day, exercising (however, because she felt so poorly, she rarely

exercised as much as she would have liked) and ritually testing her blood sugar. She continued to be upset, worried and
depressed, though, anxious that she would develop diabetes
complications, and fearing that when her blood sugar rose
(400mg%) ranges that she would run the risk of developing
diabetes ketoacidosis, or that when it was low she would be
too weak to function.

Despite both of our efforts, Mary Rose's diabetes continued its stubborn course. We, therefore, tested different types
of insulin regimens (except the insulin pump as this had
already failed) and carbohydrate counting, but her blood
sugars continued to fluctuate drastically. I could sense that
my time with her was up, and I was quite despondent, feeling
that I had been no better than all the other doctors at trying
to solve her enigmatic problem.

Then, as a last resort, I suggested we try "The Bernstein
Diet", named after its originator Dr. Richard Bernstein, who
at 40 had turned from engineer to physician, and who has
had diabetes for over 50 years. As he described in a 1992 issue
of the Medical Tribune, for years Bernstein had diabetes that
was difficult to control. It was not until he cut back on his
carbohydrate intake—to as little as 12% of his total calories—
that he could get normal blood sugars with minimal insulin
doses and eliminate his wildly fluctuating blood sugar levels.

Although I had been aware of the Bernstein Diet for many
years, I had been reluctant to recommend it because of the
high protein and high fat consumption it advocated. It is,
therefore, contrary to what is currently considered by many
authorities to be the healthiest diet: a vegetarian one high in
complex carbohydrates. The American Diabetes Association,
the American Cancer Society, Dr. Nathan Pritikin (who developed the famed Pritikin Diet, where a majority of the calories
consumed are provided by complex carbohydrates) and others have suggested that our diets should consist largely of
complex carbohydrates, and that we should lower the portion
of fats and proteins in our diet to protect against heart and
kidney disease.

However, the Bernstein Diet, with its low levels of

carbohydrates, was one "new" option that we thought was worth trying for Mary Rose. As in all aspects of life we must have an open mind, trying all options, even those not always readily accepted by the medical community. So Mary Rose began a diet that generally consisted of eggs and cheese for breakfast, fish for lunch and fish or a lean meat for dinner with plenty of fresh greens.

For Mary Rose, the Bernstein Diet has worked. Mary Rose has been able to reduce her insulin intake substantially, which has flattened out the peaks and valleys of her blood sugar level, and she is feeling much better. In her own words, "This is the best I've felt in 25 years."

Difficulty With Control: What Too Many Calories Can Do

Mr. W. is also an example of the kind of havoc too many calories from carbohydrates can wreak on diabetes control. Mr. W. was taking over 130 units of insulin and consuming around 2,500 calories with over 300 grams of carbohydrates.

This is what he has to say about his previous habit of overeating and how we treated his problem: "I think the most effective thing I have done to get my diabetes under control is to reduce the amount of food I have been eating. Previously, I was over-using insulin, because I was not keeping a diary of my calorie intake. Therefore, I allowed my intake of carbohydrates and calories to gradually increase by having additional servings and more "starchy" snacks between meals. Then, as my blood sugar levels rose, I increased my dosage of insulin to correct the situation. Now, I keep a diary, writing down everything I eat, including allowable snacks between meals and at bedtime. I note carbohydrate and calorie totals—with a target of 200 grams of carbohydrates and 1800 calories per day—along with my blood sugar levels, taken four times a day. This procedure, under the guidance of Dr. Lodewick, provided a documented record of the effect my diet was having on blood sugar levels. Consequently, my insulin dosage was gradually reduced."

As Mr. W. cut back his carbohydrate calories—even those

most people think are innocent ones like **crackers, breads and bagels**—he was able to cut his insulin dose down to less than 65 units. In addition, his blood sugar control has magnificently improved, and he feels better and feels more in control now that he better understands the relationship between food, particularly carbohydrates, and his blood sugar levels. His wife is much happier, too!

12

Measurement of Glycohemoglobin (A₁C)

Measurement of glycohemoglobin is a test that indicates how well diabetes is controlled over a 2-to-3-month period. Although I originally thought that this test might be helpful strictly from a research point of view (in terms of correlating the degree of one's diabetes control with the incidence of diabetes complications, I now find this test to be much more practical. It can be used as a diagnostic, motivative, and therapeutic tool as well. For the patient, this means increased confidence and better medical care.

Glycohemoglobin is a substance that is formed when sugar in the blood binds to the hemoglobin from red blood cells. Hemoglobin is a protein compound found within red blood cells. It delivers oxygen to body tissues and removes carbon dioxide. While hemoglobin carries out these functions, blood sugars unite with hemoglobin, forming glycohemoglobin and a fraction of this, called the hemoglobin A₁C.

Consequently, blood sugar concentration determines glycohemoglobin concentration. Also, since hemoglobin exists inside the red blood cells, and since red blood cells live 2-to-3 months or more, the concentration of glycohemoglobin can indicate what the blood sugar has been averaging over a 2-to-3-month period. Hemoglobin contained in 1-to-5-day-old red blood cells may have very little glucose attached to it, whereas hemoglobin contained in two-to three-month-old red blood cells may have many glucose molecules attached to it, especially if the blood glucose levels have been averaging very high. The different ranges for the glycohemoglobin are shown in the following table.

The above discussion sounds scientific enough, but what about the practical aspect? As I mentioned, the glycohemoglobin test can be used as a multipurpose tool. To explain its use as a diagnostic tool, I offer the following case history.

Glycohemoglobin Values*

Normal	4–8.2%
Fair Diabetes Control	8.2–9.2%
Poor Diabetes Control	9.2–18%

*As per Metpath Laboratories

Diagnostic Dilemma Solved by Glycohemoglobin

This case involves a woman in her fifties who had a history of good health but who suddenly developed an infectious illness with high temperature. She recovered from her infectious illness but then had a sudden onset of severe blurred vision, making her secretarial job impossible. Quite alarmed, she immediately sought the attention of her eye doctor (ophthalmologist), who reassured her that her eyes were fine except for some refractory changes. He suggested that diabetes might be causing the vision difficulty. Knowing that there was a history of diabetes in her family, she thought this a likely answer. She tested her urine for sugar, and sure enough, it was positive. When a blood sugar was obtained, results read 192mg%, and she called me to make an appointment as soon as possible.

Unfortunately, my office schedule was so full she could not be seen by me until several weeks later. By that time, several things had happened, she had reduced the sweets and sugar in her diet, her visual difficulties had disappeared, and her blood sugar was normal— 104mg%! With a 104mg% blood sugar, I couldn't very well make a diagnosis of diabetes, but was not sure what to make of her previous blood sugar of 192mg%. Although a value of 192mg% is high, it is not usually high enough to cause such severe blurred vision. Generally, blood sugars should be running 200-to-300mg% or more for an extended period of time before vision is affected.

To help solve this dilemma, I tested the glycohemoglobin level of this woman and sure enough, it was 9.2%, indicating that this woman did in fact have very high blood sugars and that she had had them for at least a several-week period. Although it may not initially seem encouraging for this woman to learn that her vision troubles were due to elevated blood sugars, this knowledge did solve the mystery of her vision disturbance, and she now knew what to guard against. Secondly, in the weeks preceding her visit to me, she had already proven that she could manage her diabetes by dietary control. Thirdly, she could be reassured that diabetes would cause her few complications in the future, since she had no evident diabetes complications diabetes is generally mild, and when the onset occurs in someone over the age of 50, the disease does not cause many of the major diabetes complications if good control is maintained.

Glycohemoglobin as a Motivative or Therapeutic Tool

Glycohemoglobin testing in conjunction with blood sugar testing can be a very useful tool in deciding whether or not changes in diabetes treatment are needed. Many patients come to the doctor's office maintaining that they have stuck to their diet and have been active, and indeed, their blood sugar results at the office are within acceptable range. Thus, the doctor encourages the patients to "keep up the good work."

However, it is very possible that blood sugar levels can be normal at an office visit but very abnormal later the same day. Patients often have a difficult time maintaining their diet day in and day out. The doctor knows the blood sugars are likely to get high between visits, but when a patient has acceptable blood sugars at the office, the doctor has a hard time convincing him that he ought to be more careful. This is where the glycohemoglobin test is handy. If the glycohemoglobin test result is high, then the doctor has proof that the patient could do better in maintaining good blood sugar levels. I have seen patients with glycohemoglobin levels as high as 11-to-15% who have consistently normal blood sugars on their three or four office checks per year. If the patient can have a normal blood sugar on an office visit, he should be able to get better glycohemoglobin levels. By monitoring urine sugars and/or blood sugars at home, the patient can make adjustments in diet, activity, or antidiabetic agents. In my experience, well-motivated patients such as pregnant women (who know the outcome of pregnancy depends on good control) and patients who want to minimize diabetes complications can and do normalize their glycohemoglobin levels.

In addition, this test can be used to determine whether or not patients need insulin. Although some doctors believe that all cases of diabetes can be categorized as insulin-dependent or non-insulin-dependent, it is not always that clear-cut. Some patients may benefit from insulin treatment but are not necessarily prone to ketoacidosis. If a person with diabetes is losing weight, is weak and fatigued despite proper diet, and has high glycohemoglobin levels, there is a good chance that insulin could be very beneficial.

Finally, glycohemoglobin as a guide to control can be used to evaluate diabetes control as good, fair, or poor. This distinction was previously impossible. With this diagnostic tool, correlations can be made between good diabetes control and degree of complications. Good control will correlate very highly with very few diabetes complications.

The Doctor Gets a Bad Result

After reading this chapter, you may be curious to know what *my* glycohemoglobin levels are since I have spent so much time proclaiming the value of glycohemoglobin testing. Reluctantly, I must admit that my initial glycohemoglobin result was somewhat disappointing—9.4%. After receiving this result, my competitive nature sprang into action. Not wanting to be outdone by many of my fellow insulin-dependent patients who keep their sugar levels in the normal range, I did some serious thinking.

Although in the 1970's, I tested my urine regularly with Tes-Tape, I realized that I had not regarded the positive results (which constituted 25-to-50% of my tests) as being very significant. Thinking my renal threshold was low and that Tes-Tape was extremely sensitive, I thought my blood sugars were relatively good even though I was getting positive results. Once I got my 9.4% glycohemoglobin result, however, I started testing my blood sugars more frequently at home.

Again, I must reluctantly admit that I was often getting test results of blood sugar levels between 200mg% and 320mg%, especially after breakfast. I explored this problem as I would with my patients and came to the conclusion that I was simply overeating. By cutting out the extra snacking and some of the extra portions, my blood sugars dropped toward normal—the same result my patients experience when they stop overeating. Not only that, but my glycohemoglobin dropped to 6.1%, and I succeeded in rivaling some of my better controlled diabetes patients!

Hemoglobin A₁C

More often in the 1990's, instead of the total glycohemoglobin, a fractionated glycohemoglobin, call the Hemoglobin A_1C, has been used to monitor and assess diabetes control. The Hemoglobin A_1C was used in the famed Diabetes Control and Complications trial. Discussed later in this book, the trial proved good control reduced the incidence of complications. Ideal control levels of A_1C should be under 6.2%, fair control under 8.2%, poor control is in excess of 8.2% and may go as high as 15% or more.

13

The Diabetic Diet – Food Glorious Food

There is a lot of talk about food in relation to diabetes, because it is the key to successful control of the disease. In fact, with more than half of the adult people with diabetes, diet can be the deciding factor in whether or not insulin or oral agents will be needed. Controlling excessive food intake lowers cholesterol and fat levels of the blood, which may help prevent heart and vascular disease. For people who need insulin, avoidance of overeating will prevent consistently elevated blood sugar levels, which may cause lethargy, weakness, sleep disturbance, and several other, more serious symptoms. In short, diet is crucial to proper diabetes control.

A common misconception is that diet implies either starvation or no variation whatsoever in foods eaten. I have seen many people so uninformed about the basics of diet and how it can be varied, and so concerned about keeping their blood sugars normal, that they rarely varied their diet. I knew one man, for instance, who ate the exact same breakfast, lunch, and dinner for over 30 years, because he knew it kept his blood sugar in good control. Every day, he brought a banana, a thermos of milk, and a meatball sandwich with him on the road (he worked as a traveling salesman). He cooked the meatballs the night before to assure that he got the same amount of meat with the sandwich each day. Although he certainly did a good job controlling his blood sugar and was free of any major diabetes complications, I think he could have done just as well by spicing things up a bit with a little variety! Just by knowing some basic nutritional information, food can be proportioned and varied so that ideal weight is maintained, maximal strength is assured, blood sugar is controlled, and the taste buds are satisfied!

Knowing about food and diet is not restrictive. In fact, the more you know about food, the less restrictive you have to be with your daily schedule. By knowing the approximate caloric intake of various foods, you will know how to adapt your nutritional needs to a schedule that suits you. You do not have to eat supper at 5 PM or else. You can eat at 4 PM or 8 PM or any other time as long as you know how to avoid hypoglycemia by having an appropriate snack or making adjustments in insulin doses. You can also decide which diet you prefer, taking into consideration your blood sugar, and cholesterol levels, be it vegetarian, high- or low-carbohydrate, high or low protein or high- or low-fat. When you dine at a restaurant, you'll be able to choose from a menu with greater confidence.

What is the best way to learn about proper diet? One of the worst ways is to use the so-called free diet. Too many people interpret this diet as allowing one to eat any quantity of any food that is available to munch on. With this misunderstanding, caloric intake can range from 1200-to 4000 calories, and the blood sugar can range from 40-to-1000mg%. Most people simply don't do well on unlimited calories. It is much safer to use the weighed diet or the exchange diet, both of which will be discussed in this section. By using either of these methods, you can get a good idea of the approximate caloric intake of most foods. Food labeling and calorie counting books have helped enormously in this regard and should be used as an aid to diet planning. Once you know the approximate caloric intake of the food you eat, you will be able to determine the number of calories you need to get through the day, to keep your weight ideal or get through a period of exercise. This knowledge can help you avoid the unnecessary extremes in blood sugar levels.

Before explaining in detail the exchange or weighed diet, it is vital to know that every person is different metabolically, physically, and emotionally and will thus need a different number of calories per day than another person. It is educated guesswork when a physician prescribes a certain number of calories for a patient. Two thousand calories per day may prove to be too much or too little for a particular person. In such a case, the number of calories will have to be adjusted until the proper amount is determined. This proper amount will be known when the patient has achieved ideal weight and the blood sugar levels are controlled.

Understanding a diet depends on knowing some basic facts about nutrition. Let's review some useful information about food that can help you know whether you are getting the proper daily intake of vital nutrients. The following terms will be discussed:

- gram
- calorie
- nutrient
- recommended daily allowance (RDA)
- carbohydrates
- proteins
- fats
- cholesterol
- vitamins
- fiber

A *gram* is a metric unit of weight. Approximately 30 grams equal one ounce.

A *calorie* is a measurement of energy, scientifically defined as the amount of heat needed to raise one kilogram of water one degree Centigrade. Food contains calories in the form of carbohydrate, protein, fat, and alcohol. It has been determined that there are approximately 4 calories per gram of carbohydrate, 4 calories per gram of protein, 9 calories per gram of fat, and 7 calories per gram of alcohol. With this information and with the help of the federal program which has foods labeled according to their content of carbohydrate, protein, and fat, you should be able to calculate the number of calories in anything from a water bagel to a can of soup to a Pepperidge Farm cookie, and thus incorporate a wide variety of food into your daily diet.

A *nutrient* is a substance found in food that is essential for proper bodily function. Nutrients include carbohydrates, proteins, fats, water, minerals, and vitamins. An assortment of foods each day is essential for good nutrition.

The U.S. Food and Nutrition Board has made recommendations known as the *recommended daily allowance (RDA)*,, also known as Daily Values (DV) on product packages, based on studies of nutritional requirements of healthy men and women. From these studies, the board has specified the necessary amounts of each nutrient for proper diet. It is important to remember that these recommendations are for healthy people. *Whether they are adequate for patients with poorly controlled diabetes is uncertain.*

Carbohydrates, often called the "fuel of life," are composed of three chemical elements; carbon, hydrogen, and oxygen. In an infinite number of combinations, these elements provide the major source of energy for most people of the world, particularly in Far Eastern countries, where up to 80% of the diet is carbohydrate. Grown in fields and farm lands, carbohydrates are the least expensive energy source. They provide energy to all body cells, prevent the breakdown of body muscle and fat, and regulate water and mineral balance.

There are three classes of carbohydrates. The simplest form of carbohydrate is sugar. Sugars include table sugar, cane sugar, brown sugar, honey, raw or turbinado sugars. The sugars found in fruit (fructose) and milk (lactose) are also in this group.

The second group of carbohydrates is starch. Bread, cereal, pasta, tuber vegetables (such as potatoes, carrots, and turnips), and legumes (such as peas and beans) are all starches. During digestion, these starches are converted to sugar.

Cellulose is the third carbohydrate group. Cellulose includes stalks and leaves of vegetables, fruit skins, and seeds. As the most complex group of carbohydrates, cellulose cannot be digested in the human body, but it forms the necessary bulk for proper elimination.

Proteins are nitrogen-containing compounds essential for life. They are made from simpler nitrogen-containing units called amino acids, of which there are 22 types. There are some amino acids that the human body must obtain from food because it cannot synthesize them. Essential amino acids are those that cannot be synthesized by the body.

All living cells contain protein. Protein is needed for growth, development, and tissue synthesis. It is interesting to note that insulin is a protein, as are other body hormones. The ability of the body to resist disease depends on "antibodies," which are also proteins.

The recommended minimal daily allowance of protein is 56 grams for the average man and 46 for the average woman. Athletes and muscle builders frequently consume more protein. The most common source of protein is food of animal origin: milk, meat, poultry, and fish. All these sources provide the essential amino acids for human biological processes. For the vegetarian, legumes, grains, nuts and vegetables should all be eaten daily to ensure adequate protein consumption.

Fats are a major energy source in food, containing 9 calories per gram, more than twice as many calories as carbohydrates or proteins. In America over 40% of the diet is comprised of fat. The American Diabetes Association, American Heart Association and the American Cancer Society, however, have suggested in the past few years that the amount of fat in the American diet should be reduced to probably less than 30% of the total caloric consumption, but people living with diabetes may find they need a great variety of foods so they may consume more fat than is recommended.

Fat is necessary to help transport and absorb the fat-soluble vitamins A, D, E, and K. Fats are the principal storage form of calories and are very important in providing necessary energy during strenuous exercise.

Fats include *fatty acids, triglycerides, cholesterol, and lipoprotein.* Fatty acids are long carbon and hydrogen chains, called *hydrocarbons*, ending in a carbon, oxygen, and hydrogen unit called an acid. If all the carbons in the chain are filled with hydrogen, it is called a saturated fat. If hydrogen is missing from one of the carbons in the chain, it is called a *monounsaturated fat*. If hydrogen is missing from more than one carbon in the chain, it is called a *polyunsaturated fat*. Polyunsaturated fat lowers cholesterol levels, possibly by increasing fat excretion or decreasing synthesis. Fatty acids are the energy form used by the body when glucose is not available.

Triglycerides are combinations of a compound called *glycerol* with three fatty acids. Ninety percent of the body fat is contained in this form. When the blood level of triglycerides rises above 250mg%, it is considered abnormally high, possibly a factor in heart disease.

Cholesterol is a complex combination of fatty acids and a cyclic alcohol. It contributes to the formation of body hormones, Vitamin D, and part of the bile. A high blood cholesterol level may be predisposing to heart disease. The level that is considered high and possibly dangerous is a major point of dispute among authorities. The American Heart Association now recommends that the blood cholesterol be kept under 200mg% for those under 30 years of age and under 220-to 240mg% for those less than 60. Certainly over 300mg% is high, but I have seen some healthy 80-year-old's with these levels, so no definitive statement can be made about what levels are truly dangerous, although the research literature is increasingly supporting that the level be kept under 200mg% no matter what age..

High density lipoprotein (HDL), the "good cholesterol", is a complex fat and protein substance that has been the focus of much discussion in relation to cholesterol. Although HDL transports blood cholesterol throughout the body, it is thought to prevent cholesterol from lodging in the artery walls, thus preventing hardening of the arteries (arteriosclerosis). Exercise and a high fiber diet raise the HDL blood levels.

Low density lipoprotein (LDL) is also a fat and protein complex that transports cholesterol. However, whereas HDL may

Goal	Cholesterol Total	HDL Cholesterol		LDL Cholesterol
Ideal	under 200	men over 40	women over 45	under 100
Fair	200-240	35-40	40-45	100-160
Poor	over 240	under 35	under 40	over 160

be very beneficial, LDL may, by an unknown mechanism, cause cholesterol to be released into arteries and therefore have more damaging effects, possibly accelerating arteriosclerosis. The table on the previous page summarizes what cholesterol values may mean.

Vitamins are a group of complicated substances found in small quantities in food that are vital to many bodily functions. At first, these substances were thought to be nitrogenous *(amines)*, but since that time it has been learned that few vitamins are amines. The name vitamin still remains, however. Because the body cannot synthesize most vitamins, it must depend on dietary sources. There is a major controversy over the amount of vitamins needed for proper nutrition. Dr. Linus Pauling, the Nobel Prize-winning nuclear physicist, recommended high doses of vitamin C (over 2,000mg/day!) for the prevention of the common cold. Most of the scientific community, until recently looked upon this recommendation with doubt. However, in recent years, there have been an increasing number of reports that are now suggesting that not only vitamin C but also vitamins A, E, beta-carotene, and folic acid may reduce the incidence of heart disease and cancer. Further, they may blunt the aging effects of cataract formation and arthritis. Folic acid and selenium seem to be showing good effect as disease fighters possibly preventing vascular disease. Chromium poly-nicotinate seems to have a critical role in the proper use of sugar and may help lower blood sugar levels in people—especially those with Type II diabetes. In addition, many recent studies have demonstrated that its other important effects might include raising good HDL while lowering total blood cholesterol, lowering body fat while increasing lean body muscle mass, and reversing vascular disease. It is also possible that chromium poly-nicotinate supplements might reduce body fat without dieting and improve exercise performance. It is generally believed that if there are adequate calories obtained using all the exchange lists, vitamin supplementation should not be needed, but most people don't eat right and don't get enough fresh fruits and vegetables. On the following page is a chart that lists the

	Function	Sources	RDA	AADP PAL*
Vitamin A	Important for vision, skin integrity, and gland secretions; fights infection	Green and Yellow vegetables, Fruits	4000-5000 IU	20,000 IU
Vitamin D	Regulates absorption of calcium and phosphorus from the digestive tract; essential for bone development and preservation, which will prevent fractures	Fish Milk	200-400 IU	400 IU
Vitamin E	Currently controversial, may protect red blood cells essential to cell respiration	Vegetable oils Margarine	10-20 IU	200-400 IU
Vitamin K	Necessary for blood clotting; may participate in energy transfer in tissues	Fruits Vegetables	70-140 mcg	70-140 mcg
Vitamin C (Ascorbic Acid)	Necessary for supporting tissues and for healing wounds; important for many chemical reactions in cells, including the utilization of vitamins	Fruits Vegetables	45-70 mg	500-1500 mcg
Thiamine (Vitamin B1)	Necessary for energy-generating activities, including proper use of oxygen, metabolism of glucose, and proper of glucose, central nervous system	Bran Wheat Germ Unmilled rice	1.2-2 mg	10 mg
Riboflavin (Vitamin B2)	Constituent of body enzymes involved in metabolism of carbohydrate, proteins and fat	Milk Meat Fish	1.2-2 mg	10 mg
Niacin (Vitamin B3)	Constituent of body enzymes involved in metabolism of carbohydrate, protein, and fat	Grains,Fish, Meat, Peanuts Wheat Germ	13-19 mg	100 mg
Pyridoxine (Vitamin B6)	Participates in enzyme systems necessary for carbohydrate protein, and fat metabolism	Meat Potatoes Grains	1-2 mg	6 mcg
Vitamin B12	Necessary for proper function of all cells, metabolism of nerve cells, and utilization of fat, protein, and carbohydrate	Animal protein, especially liver, muscle, meats, and dairy	3-4 mcg	12 mcg
Folic acid (Folacin)	Constituent of body enzymes needed for proper utilization of proteins and for formation of red blood cells and hemoglobin	Leafy vegetables Grains Liver	400 mcg	400 mcg

Source: Recommended Dietary Allowances, 9th Ed. Wash. DC: Food and Nutrition Board, National Research Council, (National Academy of Sciences).

*For Anti-aging and Disease Prevention: Quantities recommended by Peter A, Lodewick, M.D.

more common vitamins in terms of function, sources, and RDA as well as some recommended doses for anti-aging effect. In addition to these quantities, there are some who suggest that the following quantities may be helpful to preserve health for their anti-aging and antioxidant effect: Calcium, 1000mg; Chromium Poly-nicotinate, 200mcg; Copper, 2mg; Selenium, 200 mcg; Iron, 18mg; and zinc, 15 mg plus Boron1-2 mg; manganese, and copper in small quantities.

Over the past 10 years, the importance of *fiber* in a well-balanced and nutritionally sound diet has come to the foreground. Fiber refers to the portion of vegetarian foods that cannot be digested by the stomach and intestines. It has been recommended that adults should get at least 20 to-40 grams of plant fiber per day. Whole grain products and certain vegetables (such as peas and beans) have a high content of plant fibers. Fruits are also a source of fiber, particularly fruits that are high in pectin (such as apples). Pectin has been shown to be helpful in lowering cholesterol levels. The benefits of fiber will be elucidated in the following discussion.

Lode-A-Vits

Because of the difficulty many people have in getting quality multivitamins, I am hoping to develop a product which contains the potentially protective nutrients that are discussed in the above section.

Is there a Best Diet?

The answer to this question is very controversial. There are so many aspects that need to be addressed that is beyond the scope of this book. When insulin was first discovered in the 1920's, carbohydrate content of the diet was liberalized especially in view of the high incidence of vascular disease, associated with high blood cholesterol and triglycerides. As the 1990's approached recommendations were to make 60% of the calories come from carbohydrates, particularly complex.

However the Diabetes Control and Complications Trial (DCCT) indicates that many of the complications may come from high blood sugar. It has been the experience of many, in particular Richard Bernstein M.D. and myself that the more carbohydrates that are in the diet (even complex ones from fruits and breads) the harder it is, and the more insulin it takes, to control the blood sugar. A vicious cycle then takes place as the higher the insulin level (whether it be insulin by injection as we have seen in Type I diabetes, or the increased insulin secretion that is seen in Type II diabetes) the heavier the person gets, as insulin causes the carbohydrate to be turned into fat. It is not uncommon to see people who are on high carbohydrate diets to have high cholesterol and triglycerides and be overweight. The heavier the person the more the body fights insulin, and the more complications that result.

My experience has been that if people can maintain their weight, their blood sugar and their cholesterol on complex carbohydrate diet or vegetarian diets that is good. This would go hand in hand with the diet of Far Eastern and African countries where there is less incidence of heart and vascular disease and cancer. The high fat content of the diet may help cut down on colitis, bowel irregularity and keep the bowels moving. But for those who have problems controlling their weight, their blood sugar and lipids, diets much lower in carbohydrates may be better to achieve ideal body weight and normal blood sugars.

But before suggesting that people try to eliminate most carbohydrates from the diet, it is important to realize that fresh fruits and vegetables may have a protective effect on good health.

The medical literature seems to be increasingly supportive of the protection that vegetarians have against vascular disease and cancer. The Japanese have the lowest incidence of many forms of cancer and vascular disease in the world. But when they moved to Hawaii their cholesterol and heart attack rate goes up, and when in California their cholesterol and heart attack rate goes up even higher. Tell me it's not the

westernized diet! The same is true of many other native pop-
ulations who have low disease rates until they move into the
cities. Mention should also be made of the Seventh Day
Adventist, who do not eat meat in their diet and who have
a whopping seven year longer life span. The importance of
fresh fruits and vegetables is emphasized now by the
National Institutes of Health, the American Heart Association,
the American Cancer Society, as well as the American
Diabetes Association who are recommending at least five
servings of fresh raw fruits and vegetables per day.

Yet today very few Americans are eating enough fresh
fruits and vegetables, including myself I must reluctantly
admit. In a survey of two thousand people by the Alabama
Department of Health, just completed in 1995, it was found
that only a paltry 27% of women and 22% of men ate five
servings of fruit and vegetables. No wonder that vascular
disease, hypertension, and cancer is so prevalent! Why is this?
In my opinion, it is because in the hectic American lifestyle
where wives are working, husbands are not home, kids are
into so many sports and activities, church events, and volunteer events, that there is seldom time to prepare enough fresh
fruits and vegetables in a satisfying manner, plus the easy
access to processed foods - which may destroy some of the
essential nutrients and vitamins in food.

There is a way around this dilemma. If people are not able
to consume enough fresh fruits and vegetables - I, for one, are
one of these people as my sugar may go up if I eat to many
fruits and juices. Knowing the protective health benefits of
fresh fruits and vegetables I began using a product called
"Juice Plus." Since using this product, I have felt much more
energetic, despite working very long hours, sometimes with
minimal sleep. There must be some nutrients in the product
that I was not getting in my diet.

The product is made by a process called "flash drying",
which prevents heating and freezing from destroying the
nutrients in it that may otherwise occur when fruits and vegetables are frozen or heated. There are seventeen different
fresh fruits and vegetables in the product and it is estimated
to take several pounds of fresh fruits and vegetables to make

just one day's supply. There are no additives, and the capsule is all natural; it contains many natural vitamins, beta carotene, folic acid, ascorbic acid, live food enzymes, minerals, and fiber that are contained in fresh fruits and vegetables. And they are simple to take - two fruit capsules in the morning and two vegetable capsules in the evening.

Thus it would seem for many the best diet may be a high fiber, high-carbohydrate, and low-fat diet. But, if people have a hard time controlling their blood sugar on a high carbohydrate diet, they may possibly want to try the Bernstein diet (page 82-83) or a variation of it to even out their blood sugar excursions. The addition of a product such as Juice Plus may provide the nutrients other products may not otherwise be getting in a low carbohydrate diet.

Meal Planning with Exchange Lists or with a Weighed Diet

In 1950 a committee of representatives from the American Diabetes Association, the American Dietetic Association, and the U.S. Public Health Service published a system of diet management. The proposed diet was based on a system of food groups or lists, called exchange lists.

An exchange list consists of foods that have similar nutrient composition when used in a specified serving size. With exchanges, you can substitute one food for another within the same list. For example, one-half cup cooked string beans may be substituted for one-half cup carrots. However, a food in one exchange list should not be substituted for another; in other words, carrots should not be substituted for bacon.

When a diet is prescribed by a doctor, it is generally recommended that foods from each list be included so that all the necessary nutrients are consumed to provide energy and to regulate body functions. However, there is a profound difference in diet recommendations from diabetes specialist to diabetes specialist. Although a strict vegetarian diet may be good for many, there are many people with brittle diabetes who do not tolerate many fruits, juices, bread, bagels, and crackers as discussed earlier (especially in the Section on "Brittle Diabetes" and later in the Section on the Glycemic Index: cooked carrots may raise the blood sugar as much as regular table sugar or sucrose, calorie per calorie). For example, if a diet consisted only of meat exchanges, the vitamin C and calcium content might be inadequate, although the protein would be sufficient. Likewise, if only the bread and vegetable exchange lists were used, essential protein and vitamin B_{12} might be lacking.

Nevertheless it is important to learn about the calorie intake of foods portion per portion, and this is where the exchange lists can be helpful. By learning the protein, carbohydrate and fat content of varied foods, you will then be able to learn the total calories you eat each day and the proportion that comes from each carbohydrate, protein, and fat portion. By frequent blood sugar testing, you can then see how these different foods alter the blood sugar levels as you attempt to get as good blood sugar control as possible (ideally between 60 to 100 before meals).

Exchange lists have been recently revised so that they now emphasize the use of foods containing lower levels of fat such as skim milk and lean meat. Certain vegetables are now included with the starches. The six exchange lists are as follows:

1. **Bread.** This list includes bread, cereal, and starchy vegetables. One exchange contains 15 grams carbohydrate, 3 grams protein, and 80 calories. Several prepared foods fall into this category. Some bread exchanges are high in fiber.
2. **Meat.** This list is divided into 3 parts, lean, medium fat, and high fat meals. One exchange of lean meat (1 ounce) contains 7 grams protein, 3 grams fat, and 55 calories. Medium fat has 7 grams protein, 5 fat or 75 calories, and high fat has 7 grams protein and 8 grams fat or 100 calories. This list has been expanded, and choices can be made from meats and meat substitutes of various fat levels. Wise choices can reduce cholesterol intake.
3. **Vegetables.** One exchange contains about 5 grams carbohydrate, 2 grams protein, 2 grams fiber, and 25 calories. One exchange of a vegetable is one-half cup cooked or 120

grams. Some vegetables are more starchy and are included with the bread exchanges.

4. **Fruits.** One exchange of fruit contains 15 grams carbohydrate and 60 calories. Except for juices, fruits contain about 2 grams fiber per exchange. Serving size depends on type of fructose (fruit sugar), which varies in different fruits.

5. **Milk.** Skim milk preferred. One exchange or 8 ounces contains 12 grams carbohydrate, 8 grams protein, a trace of fat, and 80 calories. Whole milk, buttermilk, and other types of milk are also specified on the list, whole milk having 8 grams of fat or 150 calories per source and 2% having 5 grams fat or 120 calories.

6. **Fats.** One exchange of fat contains 5 grams fat and 45 calories. Here again, wise choices can be made to include polyunsaturated fats to help lower cholesterol levels.

An important thing to remember in diet planning is that your meal plan does not require many special foods or special food preparations. Foods used on the list are the same familiar foods purchased in your favorite supermarket. When you become familiar with the values that have been established for each food list and the type of food on each list, you will develop confidence in dealing with your diet. You will be able to dine at a new restaurant, the home of a friend, or even a fast-food chain operation.

A federal program was initiated in 1973 that defined procedures to be used by food companies to specify the nutritive values of foods on product labels. With the expanded knowledge of your diet, you may be able to review new products and include them in your diet. The use of specially marked dietetic products is not always necessary or even recommended.

Remember, eat a diet or food you can live with. It can be reviewed, revised, or readjusted for special conditions such as pregnancy, hypertension, or high cholesterol levels. It can be adapted to a changed lifestyle or schedule. There are diet counselors or certified diabetes educators available to help you when you need dietary advice. Use their services!

We will address the important topic of food exchange in Chapter 14. Good luck and good eating.

14

The Food Exchange List

Note: The exchanges below are based on the 1986 recommendation of the American Diabetes Association and American Dietetic Association. If there are any questions with regard to the following the correct diet, do not hesitate to ask for the expert help of a registered dietitian.

1. Bread Exchange

Each item in this list contains approximately 15 grams of carbohydrate, 3 grams of protein, a trace of fat, and 80 calories. Whole grain products average about 2 grams of fiber per serving. Some foods are higher in fiber. Those foods that contain 3 or more grams of fiber per serving are **identified with the symbol ***.

You can choose your starch exchanges from any of the items on this list. If you want to eat a starch food that is not on this list, the general rule is that:

1/2 cup of cereal, grain or pasta is one serving
1 ounce of a bread product is one serving

Your dietitian can help you be more exact.

Cereals/Grains/Pasta

*Bran cereals, concentrated	1/3 cup
*Bran cereals, flaked	1/2 cup
(such as Bran Buds™, All Bran™)	
Bulger (cooked)	1/2 cup
Cooked cereals	1/2 cup
Cornmeal (dry)	2 1/2 Tbsp.
Grapenuts	3 Tbsp.

Adapted from American Dietetic Association and American Diabetes Association.

Grits (cooked)	1/2 cup
Other ready-to-eat	3/4 cup
Unsweetened cereals	
Pasta (cooked)	1/2 cup
Puffed cereal	1 1/2 cup
Rice, white or brown (cooked)	1/3 cup
Shredded wheat	1/2 cup
*Wheat germ	3 Tbsp.

Dried Beans/Peas/Lentils

*Beans and peas (cooked)	1/3 cup
(such as kidney, white, split, blackeye)	
*Lentils (cooked)	1/3 cup
*Baked beans	1/4 cup

Starchy Vegetables

*Corn	1/3 cup
*Corn on cob, 6 in. long	1 cup
*Lima beans	1/2 cup
*Peas, green (canned or frozen)	1/2 cup
*Plantain	1/2 cup
Potato, baked	1 small (3 oz.)
Potato, mashed	1/2 cup
Squash, winter (acorn, butternut)	3/4 cup
Yam, sweet potato, plain	1/3 cup

Bread

Bagel	1/2 (1 oz.)
Bread sticks, crisp, 4 in. x 1/2 in.	2 (2/3 oz.)
Croutons, low fat	1 cup
English muffin	1/2
Frankfurter or hamburger bun	1/2 (1 oz.)
Pita, 6 in. across	1/2
Plain roll, small	1 (1 oz.)
Raisin, unfrosted	1 slice (1 oz.)
*Rye, pumpernickel	1 slice (1 oz.)
Tortilla, 6 in. across	1
White (including French, Italian)	1 slice (1 oz.)

Whole wheat   1 SLICE (1 oz.)

*3 grams or more of fiber per serving

Crackers/Snacks
Animal crackers	8
Graham crackers, 2 1/2 in. square	3
Matzoth	3/4 oz.
Melba toast	5 slices
Oyster crackers	24
Popcorn (popped, no fat added)	3 cups
Pretzels	3/4 oz.
Rye crisp, 2 in x 3 1/2 in.	4
Saltine-type crackers	6
Whole wheat crackers	2-4 slices (3/4 oz.)
no fat added (crisp breads, such as Finn™, Kavli™, Wasa™)	

Starch Foods Prepared with Fat
(Count as 1 starch/bread serving, plus 1 fat serving.)
Biscuit, 2 1/2 in. across	1
Chow mein noodles	1/2 cup
Corn bread, 2 in. cube	1 (2 oz.)
Cracker, round butter type	6
French fried potatoes, 2 in. to 3 1/2 in. long	10 (1 1/2 oz.)
Muffin, plain, small	1
Pancake, 4 in. across	2
Stuffing, bread (prepared)	1/4 cup
Taco shell, 6 in. across	2
Waffle, 4 1/2 in. square	1
Whole wheat crackers, fat added (such as Triscuits®)	4-6 (1oz.)

2. Meat Exchange
Each serving of meat and substitutes on this list contains about 7 grams of protein. The amount of fat and number of calories varies, depending on what kind of meat or substitute

you choose. The list is divided into three parts based on the amount of fat and calories: lean meat, medium-fat meat, and high-fat meat. One ounce (one meat exchange) of each of these includes:

	Carbohydrate (grams)	Protein (grams)	Fat (grams)	Calories
Lean	0	7	3	55
Medium-fat	0	7	5	75
High-fat	0	7	8	100

You are encouraged to use more lean and medium-fat meat, poultry, and fish in your meal plan. This will help decrease your fat intake, which may help decrease your risk of heart disease. The items from the high fat group are high in saturated fat, cholesterol, and calories. You should limit choices from the high-fat group to three (3) times per week. Meat and substitutes do not contribute any fiber to your meal plan.

Meats and meat substitutes that have 400 milligrams or more of sodium per exchange are indicated with this symbol*.

Lean Meat and Substitutes
(One exchange is equal to any one of the following items.)
Beef:
USDA Good or Choice grades of lean beef, such as round, sirloin, and flank steak; tenderloin; and chipped beef*.   1 oz.
Pork:
Lean pork, such as fresh ham; canned, cured or boiled ham*; Canadian bacon*, tenderloin.   1 oz.

Veal:
All cuts are lean except for veal cutlets (ground or cubed). Examples of lean veal are chops and roasts.   1 oz.

Poultry:
Chicken, turkey, Cornish hen (without skin)   1 oz.

Fish:

All fresh and frozen fish	1 oz.
Crab, lobster, scallops, shrimp, clams (fresh or canned in water*)	2 oz.
Oysters	6 med.
Tuna* (canned in water)	1/4 cup
Herring (uncreamed or smoked)	1 oz.
Sardines (canned)	2 med.

Wild Game:

Venison, rabbit, squirrel	1 oz.
Pheasant, duck, goose (without skin)	1 oz.

Cheese:

Any cottage cheese	1/4 cup
grated parmesan	2 Tbsp.
Diet cheeses* (with less than 55 calories per ounce)	1 oz.

Other:

95% fat-free luncheon meat	1 oz.
Egg whites	3 wh.
Egg substitutes with less than 55 calories per 1/4 cup	1/4 cup

400 mg or more of sodium per exchange

Medium-Fat Meat and Substitutes
(One exchange is equal to any one of the following items.)

Beef:
Most beef products fall into this category.   1 oz.
Examples are: all ground beef, roast (rib, chuck, rump), steak (cubed, Porterhouse, T-bone), and meatloaf.

Pork:
Most pork products fall into this category.   1 oz.
Examples are: chops, loin roast, Boston butt, cutlets.

Lamb:
Most lamb products fall into this category.   1 oz.
Examples are: chops, leg, and roast.

Veal:
Cutlet (ground or cubed, unbreaded)   1 oz.

Poultry:
Chicken (with skin), domestic duck or goose (well-drained of fat), ground turkey	1 oz.

Fish:
Tuna* (canned in oil and drained)	1/4 cup
Salmon* (canned)	1/4 cup

Cheese:
Skim or part-skim milk cheeses, such as:
Ricotta	1/4 cup
Mozzarella	1 oz.
Diet cheeses* (with 56-80 calories per ounce)	1 oz.

Other:
86% fat-free luncheon meat*	1 oz.
Egg (high in cholesterol, limit to 3 per week)	
Egg substitutes with 56-80 calories per 1/4 cup	1/4 cup
Tofu (2 1/2 in. x 2 3/4 in. x 1 in.)	4 oz.
Liver, heart, kidney, sweetbreads (high in cholesterol)	1 oz.

400 mg or more of sodium per exchange

High-Fat Meat and Substitutes
Remember, these items are high in saturated fat, cholesterol, and calories, and should be used only three (3) times per week.
(One exchange is equal to any one of the following items.)

Beef:
Most USDA Prime cuts of beef, such as ribs, corned beef	*1 oz.

Pork:
Spareribs, ground pork, pork sausage* (patty or link)	1 oz.

Lamb:
Patties (ground lamb)	1 oz.

Fish:
Any fried fish product	1 oz.

Cheese:
All regular cheeses*, such as American, Blue, Cheddar, Monterey, Swiss	1 oz.

Other:

Luncheon meat*, such as bologna, salami, pimento loaf	1 oz.
Sausage*, such as Polish, Italian	1 oz.
Knockwurst, smoked	1 oz.
Bratwurst*	1 oz.
Frankfurter* (turkey or chicken)	1 frank (10/lb.)
Peanut butter (contains unsaturated fat)	1 Tbsp.

Count as one high-fat meat plus one fat exchange:

Frankfurter* (beef, pork, or combination)	1 frank (10/lb.)

*400 mg or more of sodium per exchange

3. Vegetable Exchange

Each vegetable serving on this list contains about 5 grams of carbohydrate, 2 grams of protein, and 25 calories. Vegetables contain 2 to 3 grams of dietary fiber. Vegetables which contain 400 mg of sodium per serving are identified with an asterisk (*).

Vegetables are a good source of vitamins and minerals. Fresh and frozen vegetables have more vitamins and less added salt. Rinsing canned vegetables will remove much of the salt.

Unless otherwise noted, the serving size for vegetables (one vegetable exchange) is:

1/2 cup of cooked vegetables or vegetable juice
1 cup of raw vegetables

Artichoke (1/2 medium)	Mushrooms, cooked
Asparagus	Okra
Beans (green, wax, Italian)	Onions
Bean Sprouts	Pea Pods
Beets	Peppers (green)
Broccoli	Rutabaga
Brussel Sprouts	Sauerkraut*
Cabbage, cooked	Spinach, cooked
Carrots	Summer squash (crookneck)

Cauliflower   Tomato (one large)
Eggplant   Tomato/vegetable juice*
Greens (collard, mustard, turnip)
Kohlrabi Leeks   Turnips
Water chestnuts   Zucchini, cooked

* 400 mg or more of sodium

Starchy vegetables such as corn, peas, and potatoes are found on the Starch/Bread List.

4. Fruit Exchange

Each item on this list contains about 15 grams of carbohydrate and 60 calories. Fresh, frozen, and dry fruits have about 2 grams of fiber per serving. Fruits that have 3 or more grams of fiber per serving have a * symbol. Fruits juices contain very little dietary fiber.

The carbohydrate and calorie content for a fruit serving are based on the usual serving of the most commonly eaten fruits. Use fresh fruits or fruits frozen or canned without sugar added. Whole fruit is more filling than fruit juice and maybe a better choice for those who are trying to lose weight. Unless otherwise noted, the serving size for one fruit serving is:

1/2 cup of fresh fruit or fruit juice
1/4 cup of dried fruit

Fresh, Frozen, and Unsweetened Canned Fruit

Apple (raw, 2 in. across)	1 apple
Applesauce (unsweetened)	1/2 cup
Apricots (medium, raw) or	4 apricots
Apricots (canned)	1/2 cup, or 4 halves
Banana (9 in. long)	1/2 banana
*Blackberries (raw)	3/4 cup
*Blueberries (raw)	3/4 cup
Cantaloupe (5 in. across)	1/3 melon
(cubes)	1 cup
Cherries (large, raw)	12 cherries
Cherries (canned)	1/2 cup

Figs (raw, 2 in. across)	2 figs
Fruit cocktail	1/2 cup
Grapefruit (medium)	1/2 grapefruit
Grapefruit (segments)	3/4 cup
Grapes (small)	15 grapes
Honeydew melon (medium)	1/8 melon
(cubes)	1 cup
Kiwi (large)	1 kiwi
Mandarin oranges	3/4 cup
Mango (small)	1/2 mango
*Nectarine (1 1/2 in. across)	1 nectarine
Orange (2 1/2 in. across)	1 orange
Papaya	1 cup
Peach (2 3/4 in. across)	1 peach, or 3/4 cup
Peaches (canned)	1/2 cup, or 2 halves
Pear	1/2 large, or 1 small
Pears (canned)	1/2 cup or 2 halves
Persimmon (medium, native)	2 persimmons
Pineapple (raw)	3/4 cup
Pineapple (canned)	1/3 cup
Plum (raw, 2 in. across)	2 plums
*Pomegranate	1/2 pomegranate
*Raspberries (raw)	1 cup
*Strawberries (raw, whole)	1 1/4 cup
Tangerine (2 1/2 in. across)	2 tangerines
Watermelon (cubes)	1 1/4 cup

Dried Fruit

*Apples	4 rings
*Apricots	7 halves
Dates	2 1/2 medium
*Figs	1 1/2
*Prunes	3 medium
Raisins	2 Tbsp.

Fruit Juice

Apple juice/cider	1/2 cup
Cranberry juice cocktail	1/3 cup
Grapefruit juice	1/2 cup

Grape juice	1/3 cup
Orange juice	1/2 cup
Pineapple juice	1/2 cup
Prune juice	1/3 cup

*3 or more grams of fiber per serving

5. Milk Exchange

Each serving of milk or milk products on this list contains about 12 grams of carbohydrate and 8 grams of protein. The amount of fat in milk is measured in percent (%) of butterfat. The calories vary, depending on what kind of milk you choose. The list is divided into three parts based on the amount of fat and calories: skim/very lowfat milk, lowfat milk, and whole milk. One serving (one milk exchange) of each of these includes:

	Carbohydrate (grams)	Protein (grams)	Fat (grams)	Calories
Skim/Very Lowfat	12	8	trace	90
Lowfat	12	8	5	120
Whole	12	8	8	150

Milk is the body's main source of calcium, the mineral needed for growth and repair of bones. Yogurt is also a good source of calcium. Yogurt and many dry or powdered milk products have different amounts of fat. If you have questions about a particular item, read the label to find out the fat and calorie content.

Milk is good to drink, but it can also be added to cereal and to other foods. Many tasty dishes such as sugar-free pudding are made with milk (see the Combination Foods list). Add life to plain yogurt by adding one of your fruit servings to it.

Skim and Very Lowfat Milk

skim milk	1 cup
1/2 % milk	1 cup
1% milk	1 cup
lowfat buttermilk	1 cup
evaporated skim milk	1/2 cup
dry nonfat milk	1/3 cup
plain nonfat yogurt	8 oz.

Lowfat Milk

2% milk	1 cup fluid
plain lowfat yogurt (with added nonfat milk solids) 8 oz.	

Whole Milk

The whole milk group has much more fat per serving than the skim and lowfat groups. Whole milk has more than 3 1/4% butterfat. Try to limit your choices from the whole milk group as much as possible.

whole milk	1 cup
evaporated whole milk	1/2 cup
whole plain yogurt	8 oz.

6. Fat Exchange

Each serving on the fat list contains about 5 grams of fat and 45 calories.

The foods on the fat list contain mostly fat, although some items may also contain a small amount of protein. All fats are high in calories and should be carefully measured. Everyone should modify fat intake by eating unsaturated fats instead of saturated fats. The sodium content of these foods varies widely. Check the label for sodium information.

Unsaturated Fats

Avocado	1/8 medium
Margarine	1 tsp
*Margarme, diet	1 Tbsp.
Mayonnaise	1 tsp.
*Mayonnaise, reduced-calorie	1 Tbsp.

Nuts and Seeds:

Almonds, dry roasted	6 whole
Cashews, dry roasted	1 Tbsp.
Pecans	2 whole
Peanuts	20 small or 10 large
Walnuts	2 whole
Other nuts	1 Tbsp.
Seeds, pine nuts, sunflower (without shells)	1 Tbsp.
Pumpkin seeds	2 tsp.

Oil (corn, cottonseed, safflower, soybean, sunflower, olive, peanut)	1 tsp.
*Olives	10 small or 5 large
Salad dressing, mayonnaise-type	2 tsp.
Salad dressing, mayonnaise-type, reduced-calorie	1 Tbsp.
*Salad dressing (all varieties)	1 Tbsp.
*Salad dressing, reduced-calorie	2 Tbsp.

(Two tablespoons of low-calorie salad dressing is a tree food.)

Saturated Fats

Butter	1 tsp.
*Bacon	1 slice
Chitterlings	1/2 ounce
Coconut, shredded	2 Tbsp.
Coffee whitener, liquid	2 Tbsp.
Coffee whitener, powder	4 tsp.
Cream (light, coffee, table)	2 Tbsp.
Cream, sour	2 Tbsp.
Cream (heavy, whipping)	1 Tbsp.
Cream cheese	1 Tbsp.
*Salt pork	1/4 ounce.

*If more than one or two servings are eaten, these foods have 400 mg. or more of sodium.
**400 mg. or more sodium per serving.

There are some foods that you won't find on the exchange lists. Salt, pepper, herbs, spices, parsley, lemon, horseradish, vinegar, mustard, celery salt, onion salt, or powder, garlic, and bottled hot pepper sauce are all flavor bonuses with a "free" exchange rating. Diet calorie free beverages, tea, coffee, nonfat bouillon, unsweetened gelatin, and unsweetened pickles are free, too.

Also, there are quick energy foods containing sugar that may be needed from time to time to treat low sugar reactions or prevent them. A list of these foods with the approximate amount of sugar in each follows:

QUICK ENERGY FOOD LIST

Food	Portion	Bread Exchange	Fat Exchange	Fruit Exchange
Date bar	1 (2x1-inch)	1/2	1	
Animal crackers	8	1		
Nabisco sugar wafers	6	1	1	
Chocolate covered grahams	2	1	1	
Creme wafer sticks	3	1	1	
Fig Newton Cakes	2	1		
Oatmeal cookies	1 1/2	1		
Old-fashioned ginger snaps	3	1		
Oreo creme sandwich	2	1	1	
Vanilla wafers	5	1		
Apple Danish coffee cake 14 oz.	1/8	1/2	2	1

The chart on page 130 is a guide showing the approximate number of each of the various exchanges that might be included in the daily diet. Note that the number of exchanges varies according to the daily caloric intake that is allowed. The figures have been rounded to the nearest whole number. Other arrangements are possible, and plans may be modified to suit individual preferences or needs. In general, the exchanges should be spread out in three to six meals. Three is better for the non-insulin-dependent people with diabetes, and six is better for the insulin-dependent people with diabetes.

Remember, Pritikin and Anderson recommend that 60 to 80% of total calories, come from complex carbohydrates; the American Diabetes Association suggests 50 to 60% come from carbohydrates; whereas Bernstein and other physicians claim that better diabetes control can be obtained only with a much lesser amount, perhaps 40% or less, coming from carbohydrates. Time, experience, knowledge of foods, blood sugar testing and maybe the help of a registered dietitian will be important to help you learn what foods are best for you.

Calories	Carbohydrate (GMS.)	Percent of total cal.	Protein (GMS.)	Percent of total cal.	Fat (GMS.)	Percent of total cal.	List 1 Bread	List 2 Meat	List 3 Veg.	List 4 Fruit	List 5 Milk	List 6 Fat
800	106	53%	45	19%	25	28%	3	4	2	3	1/2	1
1000	127	51%	55	22%	30	27%	5	4	2	2	1	2
1200	142	47%	65	23%	40	30%	6	5	2	2	1	3
1500	199	53%	76	20%	45	27%	7	5	2	4	2	4
1800	214	48%	96	22%	60	30%	9	7	2	3	2	5
2000	264	53%	98	20%	60	27%	9	7	3	6	2	5
2200	279	51%	108	20%	70	29%	10	8	3	6	2	6
2400	311	52%	121	20%	75	28%	11	8	4	6	3	7
2600	326	50%	131	21%	85	29%	12	9	4	6	3	8
2800	353	51%	152	20%	95	29%	14	10	4	7	4	9

This table provides information on daily food plans with exchanges. **Note:** The average carbohydrate is 48-53%, protein 20-23%, fat 27-30%, in these exchanges. As you become more familiar with them you may want to change the calories and percentages as you become aware of what is best for you as far as weight, blood sugar and blood cholesterol. Work with your doctor and dietitian.

15

How to Use the Exchange Diet System

For Type II Non-Insulin Dependent Diabetes

Suppose you have a weight problem along with your diabetes, and your doctor prescribes a diet of approximately 1200 calories. Because this particular doctor is hard pressed for time, he simply gives you a diet list, wishes you luck, directs you to the exit door, and expects you to know what to do from there. This lack of explanation may mean the end of the diet (and understandably so!) before it ever begins. If the doctor fails to do the logical thing, which is to enlist the help of a registered dietitian, or a certified diabetes educator (CDE), or if you decide not to do so yourself, the chart on the previous page can help you figure out an appropriate diet.

However, now that you understand more about nutrition and food exchanges, you can take the bull by the horns, gather relevant information, and create your own meal plan within the limits your doctor has outlined for you. Using the exchange chart on the previous page, you will find that for a 1200-calorie diet you are allowed the following exchanges: 1 milk, 2 vegetable, 2 fruit, 6 bread, 5 meat, and 3 fat. By checking your cupboards, refrigerator and wallet, you can choose the foods that are most appealing to you when designing your diet. You can satisfy the hunger and create wonderful meals that are allowed by your physician and incorporates the exchanges you are allowed. Your plan might look something like the table on the next page.

You will notice that this sample meal plan provides no between-meal snacks. Theoretically, it may be better to eat nutritional snacks between meals and eat less food for breakfast, lunch, and dinner so that less insulin from the pancreas is required at any given time to assimilate the food. However, by eating between the three traditional daily meals, there is further titillation of the taste buds, and there is a greater chance of succumbing to the deadly sin of gluttony. Therefore, if you have a difficult time controlling your appetite, three meals per day may be preferable.

	Milk	Vegetable	Fruit	Bread	Meat	Fat
Breakfast	1-1/3 cup with cereal		1-1/4 cup strawberries	40 grams or 1-1/3 ounce	1/2 cup cottage	
Lunch	iced tea	lettuce		Bran Buds 2 slices rye bread	cheese 2 ounces or 60 grams ham	1 tsp mayonnaise
Dinner		salad and 1/2 cup beets mushrooms	1/3 cantaloupe (260 grams)	1/3 cup corn (80 grams) 1/2 cup beans	3 ounces hamburger	1 tsp salad dressing

Once you are on your diet for a given length of time (say between 4 to-6 weeks), you will know whether you are succeeding by checking your weight and blood sugar. Depending on how well you are faring, you can add or subtract 100-to-300 calories from your daily intake for another 4 to-6 week period. Remember: Patience and "stick-to-it-iveness" provide a winning strategy. Quick-loss fad diets have had little lasting success. Weight loss takes time, since it took time for your unwanted pounds to accumulate. Stick to it, and don't become frustrated!

This brings me to one final point. What happens if you do succumb and eat some tempting delicacy, or, as my patients say: "cheat"? When this happens, I implore you not to give up, for you are not alone. In fact, you are probably in the majority. In my experience with diabetes, I know very few people who do not slip off their diet from time to time. The major point is to be as conscientious as you can without giving up if your willpower takes a temporary nose dive. One splurge in and of itself will not smash your progress and goals.

I know one person who actually sets aside a certain time during the week to snack on a particular goodie. By this controlled indulgence (the words are not necessarily mutually exclusive!) you may be more likely to stick to your diet during the rest of the week. Dieting is not a punishment! Instead, it is self-awareness and modification of habits for a healthier you. Once you understand the exchange system, you may want to try other nutritional options.

For Type I Insulin-Dependent Diabetes

If you require insulin injections for diabetes control, you can use diet guidelines similar to those described for the non-insulin-dependent diabetes. There are a few distinctions, however. While the non-insulin dependent people with diabetes can usually choose between three moderate or six light meals per day, it is better for you to eat the six smaller meals per day, so that there is not such a time lapse between meals, especially when you are active. A non-insulin-dependent people with diabetes can often skip meals without seriously risking hypoglycemia, but if you, as an insulin-dependent people with diabetes, skip meals, the risk of hypoglycemia is much greater. If you do find that you can skip a meal without developing hypoglycemia, it may be because your blood glucose is very high at the time so that it takes several hours to reduce it to normal levels. Although skipping a meal may help normalize blood levels, it is much better not to have elevated blood sugar in the first place!

Another major problem you may experience is reducing your caloric intake when you are taking so much insulin. I have often seen insulin-dependent people with diabetes consume way too many calories and then take a large dose of insulin to keep the blood glucose from getting exceedingly high. Then, when the doctor says to cut back on the calories, the patient will complain that when he does so, he feels weak and uncomfortable. The explanation is that the patient is suffering from hypoglycemia due to the calorie cutback while he is still taking a relatively large amount of insulin.

If you have been in a similar predicament, the best thing to do is cut back on calories gradually (perhaps by 100 calories or so every two to three days) while at the same time gradually reducing your insulin dose (maybe by two to four units at a time). This is another situation where home blood sugar monitoring is a useful guide in determining how much to decrease the calories and insulin dose without developing hypoglycemia. Your doctor should be able to answer any questions you may have about modification of calorie intake or insulin dose.

16

Distilled Water: The Healthiest Water

One of my favorite escapes is to get away to the Adirondack Mountains in upstate New York, where the forests and lakes are of unparalleled beauty. In times gone by, I've often stopped at Big Wolf Lake or one of the other crystal-clear lakes after a brisk hike or jog, just to take a sip of the pristine water—never worrying about chemicals or pollutants. I wouldn't be so sure about that these days. Today, even our everyday drinking water is a suspect.

For those of us with diabetes, the quality of our drinking water is an important matter to consider. Just as we are concerned about the food we eat, so should we be about the water we drink. We should be drinking water that is as pure as possible. There have been repeated reports that bacteria and chemicals can be very serious and even life threatening. In June 1995, the Centers for Disease Control and Prevention and the Environmental Protection Agency expressed concern that, although tap water may be safe for many healthy people, it may be dangerous for those with weakened immune systems. They most likely were concerned about AIDS victims, but certainly people with complicated and uncontrolled diabetes might also be susceptible to some infectious agents formed in tap water.

Most of our drinking water comes from public water systems or from private wells, both of which are treated with chemicals to control their level of contamination. However, impurities still exist along with the additive chemicals. Rain water is not entirely free of "impurities," either, often containing a considerable amount of chemicals acquired as rain falls through polluted air (a phenomenon called "acid rain," which has recently been identified as a potent environmental hazard).

This rain water, in turn, can taint water beds, springs and streams.

Even the much-touted mineral water may contain certain minerals, metals and inorganic compounds that the body can't use, and that may have an adverse effect on those of us with diabetes. Even the expensive bottled mineral water and the water supply in some communities are considered "hard" water, because they naturally contain higher levels of minerals such as lime, calcium, magnesium, iron, and silicon nitrates than regular or "soft" water (if you regularly find a soap-scum rim around the bathtub after a bath or shower, you live in a community with a hard water supply; the scum forms because mineral-laden water cannot dissolve substances well, so some of the minerals combine with the soap and precipitate into a grainy scum).

Although the body does require a certain amount of these minerals, frequent imbibing of water with a high mineral content can be too much of a good thing. Calcium and other minerals can deposit in heart chambers or valves and arteries, causing "hardening of the arteries" or arteriosclerosis. This is a disease characterized by thickening of blood vessel walls. Left unchecked, arteriosclerosis affects normal blood flow and can lead to a heart attack or stroke. When it affects arteries in the legs, arteriosclerosis can cause a great deal of pain and can lead to eventual limb loss due to the reduced supply of oxygen. It is therefore vitally important to prevent the formation of these deposits so that we do not add to the stress on our bodies that diabetes already exerts.

On top of that, water supplies contain a number of chemicals that are either added to the water (like chlorine to limit germs or fluoride to limit dental decay) or that flow into water supplies from the ground (these would be organic substances like lithium, arsenic, radium, and cobalt). I would speculate that these "pollutants" are not always healthful, and may best be avoided. A report in *Newsweek*, March 21, 1994, states that chemical pollutants in waters may contain some chemicals that have an adverse, estrogen-like effect, something most men would like to avoid.

The only type of water that seems to be fit for consumption is distilled water, which is water that is absolutely free of any minerals or chemicals. Distilled water is made pure by first being heated to the point of vaporization, so that all the "impurities" are left behind. Then, the water vapor is condensed. This process results in water that is in its purest form. Distillation is the single most effective method of water purification.

In addition to the benefit of being pollutant-free, distilled water is an excellent solvent. It is possible, therefore, that it could dissolve mineral deposits that have accumulated on artery walls. Distilled water might also dissolve the mineral deposits that often lodge in tissues as one gets older, thereby partially reversing the arthritis and joint disease that these mineral deposits cause.

Thus, for those of us with diabetes, drinking distilled water would seem to be especially important since most diabetes complications are a result of the accelerated aging effects of diabetes. So, we experience the early onset of such age-related problems as joint and vascular disorders. Thus, if the supposed benefits of distilled water are found to be scientifically sound, then drinking it would be of great benefit to those of us with diabetes in helping to ward off the disease's premature aging effects.

There is some evidence to suggest that distilled water may be more healthy than regular tap or mineral water. For example, Dr. Allen E. Banik, an optometrist from Nebraska who passed away at the ripe old age of 87, studied the water-drinking habits of three communities: Hunza, a village in the Himalayas; Vilcabab in Ecuador, South America and Abkhazia in southern Russia—all areas where the people are known for their long lifespans. The people of these towns are also known to be more vigorous in their old age than the elderly in most modern societies. The one common trait that could explain the longevity of the people in these three communities was the type of water they drank. The water source in each of these villages was composed of glacier water, which, through nature's filtering process, is as pure as distilled water. (You can read more about these communities in *National Geographic*, 143:93, January 1973). Subsequently, Banik's research inspired him to pen the book, *Your Water and Your Health*, published in 1990 by Keats Publishing, Inc.

Another interesting phenomenon related to distilled water is French wine. The French are known for their high fat diet, yet they are less prone to vascular disease than people in other western countries. Some preliminary evidence surprisingly points to wine—a form of natural grape distilled water—a part of every French meal, imparting some kind of protective effect.

Then, there is the anecdotal evidence of Dr. Brown Landone, a neurologist from Nebraska, who was a close friend of Dr. Banik's. At the age of 17, Dr. Landone had been told that he would die within months from calcification of his heart valves. With nothing to lose, he decided to start drinking distilled water. Dr. Landone subsequently survived to the ripe old age of 98. Although this phenomenon cannot be directly attributed to the distilled water he drank, I would guess that it may have, somehow, contributed to his longevity. Another remarkable story is that of Captain Diamond (a patient of Dr. Landone's), who was crippled with arthritis and had become bedridden by the age of 70. After a consultation with Dr. Landone, he began drinking only distilled water. Shortly thereafter, Captain Diamond was teaching class at age 76, participated in a walk from Sacramento to New York at the age of 103, and at age 110 attended a function where he danced all night with a 16-year-old-girl. He finally died when he was 120 years old.

In the medical community, the use of distilled water to prevent the mineral deposits that can block kidney dialysis machines is well known. These mineral plugs are purged by running distilled water through the dialysis tubes, thereby restoring these machines to their normal function of cleansing the blood of patients with kidney failure.

These are just some speculations on the health benefits of distilled water. Although more scientific, documented evidence is needed to corroborate some of the findings and fact-based anecdotal accounts I've mentioned, I am so intrigued by the possible value of distilled water that I now have a water distiller in my home, hoping that any adverse effects from 28 years of diabetes may be reversed, and potential problems in the future prevented. And I am excited about the possibility.

Resource: US EPA Safe Drinking Water Hotline (1-800-426-4791)

17

Weight Loss

Eat little and avoid sweets.
—LEO TOLSTOY IN HIS "TEN RULES OF LIFE"

No one ever regrets having eaten too little
.   —THOMAS JEFFERSON

How to get thin— do not eat bread, cake, potatoes, rice, cream, butter,
milk, pastries, sweets, fats, minces, puddings, stews, salt meats, fish,
or anything containing starch or sugar!
                                                     –GENERAL GEORGE PATTON

In 50% of the cases of overweight people with diabetes, weight loss is critical in controlling diabetes. For many people, especially with Type II Diabetes, shedding excess pounds will help lower blood sugars to normal levels or at least improve them enough so that insulin or oral agents may not be necessary. Yet many patients faced with a weight problem say despondently, "All I have to do is look at food and I gain weight." Many of these patients will go to their doctors with their weight problems and will be accused of not following their diet correctly, with the implication that they are lying if they say they do. As a result, they become further depressed with their lack of results (as well as with their looks) and give up completely.

The reasons why some patients have so much difficulty losing weight are complex. It is probably true that some people can eat more than others and not have a weight problem. For instance, women patients sometimes say, "My husband eats twice as much as I do and he is as skinny as a rail." The explanation for this probably lies in the difference in body chemistry and hormones, but medical research still has no definitive explanation.

Be this as it may, how do patients lose weight? With the low-carbohydrate diet many patients lose weight. This diet has been promulgated by Drs. Robert Atkins and Richard K. Bernstein. Here the low carbohydrates result in lower insulin levels or requirement. The lower the insulin level, the less the fat. To replace the carbohydrates not seen in the diet, the body uses its own calories from the breakdown in fats – referred to as "The Fat Burning Diet". But they must be sure they are getting the needed nutrients that are thought to protect vegetarians from disease. The plant chemicals found in fresh fruits and vegetables can be replaced with the addition of vitamins and/or the use of JuicePlus which contains extracts from many pounds of fresh fruits and vegetables without sugar content. This is an important addition to such low carbohydrate diets. Once the weight is down, the fat is gone, and the blood sugars normal, gradual resorption of carbohydrates in the diet may be possible – especially if significant exercise is begun. To learn more details on these diets, listen to the Richard Bernstein tapes, Bernstein Plan Type 1 and Bernstein Plan Type 2 available through PRANA Publications (1-800-735-3726) and Dr. Eaden Book, Protein Power, also through PRANA Publications.

One lady who has tried a low carbohydrate diet after years of poor control on a high carbohydrate diet writes, "I have been on the high protein diet for 2 months. I have virtually eliminated breads, starches, fresh fruits, and juices from my diet and for the first time in years my blood sugars are under control. They range from 70-160, the 160 being 2 hours after a meal. I feel better than I have in years and have much more energy." *Georganne Dewberry*, July 8, 1996.

To lose weight, people must consume fewer calories than their bodies burn. They must determine the optimum number of calories per day that will cause a weight loss. They must then adhere as closely as possible to that figure.

The realization that obesity is not just a cosmetic problem, but a health problem as well, is the another step toward a successful weight loss program. Weight Watchers and Overeaters Anonymous are two organizations that have been very successful in overcoming the psychological barriers of losing weight. Psychoanalysis, psychotherapy, and hypnosis are expensive alternatives that may also be helpful. Behavior modification has also become popular for many patients with weight problems. This program identifies several situations and moods for which the response of overeating has become almost automatic. Watching television, working in the kitchen, attending social events, and being bored or depressed after a long day are factors that frequently cause overeating. By keeping a diary of daily events and connecting these events to food eaten, patients may learn what prompts them to overeat, and they may learn to avoid the circumstances that trigger the overeating.

Knowledge of caloric and nutrient value of foods is also a great aid in weight control. Many patients are unaware of the number of calories contained in the foods they eat. Sweets are frequently higher in fat calories than in sugar calories. Nuts, seeds, crackers, and fried foods are especially high in calories because of their fat content. It is important, then, to limit the intake of these high-fat foods as well as those containing sugar calories, especially when significant carbohydrates are taken into the diet. Another recourse to those who are not able to control their overeating is the use of appetite suppressants. Many bariatrics physicians (physicians who specialize in weight loss) often recommend them to people who have lost good amounts of weight only to gain it right back again (the famous yo-yo syndrome). My experience has been very good with many people keeping weight off with the help of these suppressants. Overeaters should discuss this with their doctor. Finally, there are a number of other medications that look promising for the future. They may work to prevent fat absorption so that the calories eaten are not absorbed. Weight loss and improved blood sugars will result with these medications.

As will be discussed in one of the next chapters, another strategy to help shed those extra pounds is to make the body burn more calories; in other words, exercise more. If the body burns an extra 500 calories per day, half a pound or more per week will be lost.

Marathoners exemplify the art of weight control. Besides exercising regularly, they tend to follow more nutritious diets, eliminating "junk" food and desserts. This high-exercise, low junk-food regimen certainly seems to pay off, for it is very rare to see an overweight marathoner.

18

The Glycemic Index and the Sweet Tooth

To eat or not to eat: that is the question...

In the summer of 1983, an article in one of the most prestigious medical journals, *The New England Journal of Medicine*, indicated that plain sugar caused no more of a rise in blood sugar than did an equal caloric equivalent of potato or wheat starch. The daily newspapers interpreted this to mean that some people with diabetes can eat sugar. This was very welcome news indeed for those people with diabetes who have the same weakness as nondiabetics for foods that have been made especially enticing by the addition of various sugars or sweeteners.

The medical community, however, was stunned, having long believed in the value of distinguishing between simple and complex carbohydrates. The simple sugars include sucrose, glucose, and fructose, all of which cause an immediate rise in blood sugar and fructose which may not cause as much of a rise. Complex sugars contained in potatoes and whole grain bread cause a much lower rise in blood sugar. Well, *The New England Journal of Medicine* article was not the only one to bring this dogma into doubt. Other recent studies have reached similar conclusions, indicating that foods of equal caloric value may have differing tendencies to raise blood sugar, but that this tendency was not based on whether a food was composed of simple or complex carbohydrates. This tendency foods have of raising blood sugar levels is measured by a system now referred to as the "glycemic index," which uses glucose as the food against which all others are measured, since glucose has the greatest tendency to raise blood sugar.

Some foods with their "glycemic" blood sugar responses appeared in an article in *American Health* (January-February 1984) and are shown on the next page. As you can see from this chart, fructose, the simple sugar found in many fruits and vegetables, has a relatively low glycemic index, causing much less of a rise in blood sugar than equivalent calories in potato or cereal. Peanuts also produce a very low blood sugar response, although their large fat content makes them a snack to be wary of, especially if body weight and blood cholesterol are problems.

Which foods boost insulin levels? This lists shows how quickly different foods boost blood sugar and raise your insulin. Foods with a high number act the most like glucose, leading to an insulin jump. Foods with a low index give a slow rise in blood sugar; for example fructose, fruits and complex carbohydrates.

Honey and Sugars

Fructose	20	Honey	87
Sucrose	59	Glucose	100

Bread, Pasta, Corn, and Rice

Wholewheat spaghetti	42		
Brown rice	66		
White spaghetti	60	White bread	69
Sweet corn	59	Wheat bread	72
		White rice	72

Breakfast Cereals

Oatmeal	49	Shredded Wheat	67
All-Bran	51	Cornflakes	80

Fruits

Apples	39	Bananas	62
Oranges	40	Raisins	64
Orange juice	46		

Root Vegetables

Sweet potatoes	48	White potatoes	70

| Yams | 51 | Carrots | 92 |
| Beets | 64 | Parsnips | 97 |

Dairy Products

| Skim milk | 32 | Ice Cream | 36 |
| Whole milk | 34 | Yogurt | 36 |

Peas and Beans

Soybeans	15	Chickpeas	36
Lentils	29	Lima beans	36
Kidney beans	29	Baked beans	40
Black-eyed peas	33	Frozen peas	51

Odd and Ends

Peanuts	13	Sponge cake	46
Sausages	28	Potato chips	51
Fish sticks	38	Pastry	59
Tomato Soup	38	Mars bar	68

This brings up some crucial points, for these studies knock at the very foundation of the ADA exchange system that has been recommended for years. They may, however, help to explain why some people with diabetes have found their blood sugar 120 mg% on one day and 240 mg% the next, frustrated by the fact that they had not "cheated" on their exchange diets; the answer may lie in their having eaten foods of the same caloric value but differing glycemic index value, e.g., an apple versus a banana, orange juice versus an orange.

These studies also seem to conflict somewhat with the high-fiber, low-fat diets of Nathan Pritikin and James Anderson, M D., as some studies have shown that whole wheat bread tends to cause more of a rise in blood sugar than does ice cream. The diet and exercise programs of Pritikin and Anderson have helped many people with diabetes and vascular disorders. However, while these diets curtail a great deal of fat, and while it may be that the fat and total caloric intake of the average American is more detrimental than the sugar intake in and by itself, it is also very possible that people with diabetes do not have to be quite as restrictive of the simple carbohydrates as Pritikin and Anderson recommend as long as the blood sugar is being kept under good control!!

Finally, this brings up a key question that is constantly being bandied about among people in the health fields: Should people with diabetes eat sweets? There are some foods with sweeteners that have no calories in them, such as cyclamate, saccharin, and aspartame, which is derived from protein. These should have little effect on blood sugar and therefore should be able to be consumed in moderation. Reasons not to consume them might be the taste, especially bitter in saccharin, and the cost. (Aspartame sweeteners tend to be higher in cost.) There is some concern that cyclamate and saccharin may cause cancer, but studies that have been done over the past 10 years have not shown an increased incidence of cancer in saccharin users. Average consumption of such sweeteners is probably quite safe.

As for the caloric sweeteners, there are several on the market. They may contain table sugar (sucrose), glucose (dextrose), fructose (fruit sugar), or sorbitol. (Sorbitol is closely related in composition to glucose and fructose.) The amount of sorbitol a person can eat is probably somewhat limited, because an excessive amount causes a disturbing bout of diarrhea. Regardless, care should be taken not to overdo any of these sweets.

While it is probably quite true that cake or candy will not cause more of a rise in blood sugar than an equal number of calories from white potato or bread, it is also true that especially rich cake, such as Chocolate Mousse de Quoi, frequently has extra calories from butter, fat, or protein, so that the intake has to be a very small quantity in order to avoid going overboard. There are not many mortals who can limit themselves to such a minuscule portion of such an enticing sweet. The temptation to overindulge is simply too great, even for well-disciplined people with diabetes, and especially if they are placing too much confidence in the new glycemic index theory. People who must watch their caloric intake to keep their weight, as well as blood sugar, down might also be tempted to sacrifice nutritious foods just to have that high-calorie piece of cake. By eating sweets from table sugar, more insulin is needed to keep the blood sugar normal, and insulin per se may further provoke the appetite and then more overeating, thus setting up a vicious cycle. If, despite all good intentions, they are still inclined to incorporate a small amount of sweets in their diet, it is imperative to test their blood sugars to see the response. They may especially want to try some confections that are made with fructose to prove for themselves what many of the studies alluded to above seem to have shown (i.e., that fructose has a low glycemic index).

People with Type II diabetes who suffer from overweight and high blood insulin levels should be particularly interested in how the body responds to various types of sugars. As reported by Dr. Judith Rodin, professor of psychology at Yale, in the January-February 1984 issue of *American Health*, fructose may not stimulate the appetite as much as glucose. In her study, she found that when volunteers were given a drink with 192 calories from fructose in it, they subsequently ate much less compared to volunteers who were given a 192-calorie glucose drink. She believes that occurs because fructose has much less of a triggering effect on blood insulin and consequently on the appetite.

Conclusion and Recommendation

Recent studies have surprised many by indicating that foods of the same caloric value provoke different levels of blood sugar, due to variations in their "glycemic indices." Ice cream, for example, may cause a lower rise in blood sugar than does whole wheat bread. Despite these recent findings, I would be cautious about indulging in sweets for the above-explained reasons. And I would definitely continue to rely on blood sugar testing, keeping in mind that the ideal goal is to keep the blood sugar as close to the 60-to-120 mg% range as possible. If sugars are not staying in these ranges, the low carbohydrate diet of Bernstein or a modification of it may be very helpful – see previous discussions!

19

The Power of Exercise

SOCRATES: And is not bodily habit spoiled by rest and idleness, but preserved for a long time by motion and exercise?
—PLATO, Theaetetus

Certain health leaders of medicine have been debating the value of exercise in promoting overall well-being. Questions still exist in the minds of some over the benefits of exercise in preventing heart attacks, hypertension, and strokes. Diabetes has not been free of this controversy. In fact, for many years, exercise for the person with diabetes was considered by many physicians to be strictly verboten. Children with diabetes were considered sickly and were pampered and isolated from their sportsminded friends. The psychological consequences of this attitude included depression and rebellion. Fortunately, there has been a shift in attitude during recent years, and the value of exercise in diabetes care has been more fully recognized.

We owe thanks to people like Bill Talbert, the outstanding U.S. champion tennis professional, who has been taking insulin since shortly after its discovery in the 1920's. The hockey player, Bobby Clarke, who developed diabetes at age 14, went on to score over 1000 points in the National Hockey League and was voted Most Valuable Player several times. Other sports stars with diabetes include Jackie Robinson, Catfish Hunter, and Ron Santo. Thanks to these great athletes, we know that exercise need not be eliminated or curtailed from a diabetes' lifestyle. People with diabetes can be highly capable of strenuous exercise and outstanding sports achievements. This is no more evident than in the stellar performance of Pete Powers (now a physician), who has had diabetes since age 14 and has the distinction of running a marathon in a speedy 2 hours and 42 minutes! Also, Tim Belknap who served as Mr. Universe in 1985.

Nowhere in medicine is the effect of exercise as profound as it is in diabetes. Particularly in insulin-dependent people with diabetes, exercise can have a dramatic effect in lowering blood sugar levels if the diabetes is well controlled. In many camps for children with diabetes, exercise is heavily empha- · sized and it has been found the average insulin dose can often be cut in half with no change in diet as a result. Although the effect of exercise may differ somewhat between the Type I insulin-dependent and Type II non-insulin-dependent children with diabetes, exercise usually allows more liberal eating while maintaining normal blood sugar levels.

Exercise for People with Type I Insulin-Dependent Diabetes

Since Type I insulin-dependent diabetes creates a dysfunctional insulin system, exercise allows a decrease in insulin requirement and may help to avoid the possibility of hypoglycemia. This is especially true for whose pancreas secretes little or no insulin.

In the person without diabetes, the blood insulin level drops with exercise, thereby allowing blood sugar levels to remain within normal range without low blood sugar. In Type I diabetes, the blood insulin level depends on the amount and type of insulin injected and the rate at which it is absorbed. In addition, the absorption rate of insulin may depend on the type of exercise and the site of injection; i.e., whether the site is the arm, stomach, or leg. At rest insulin is absorbed more quickly in the arm than in the leg. However, when the legs are used in exercise, insulin is absorbed more quickly, and if insulin is injected there, it may have a more pronounced effect on the blood sugar level, possibly leading to an insulin reaction.

Exercise not only promotes more rapid absorption of insulin at the injection site, but also enhances the effect of insulin. These factors have to be considered when planning exercise in order to prevent blood sugar levels that are too high or too low. In addition, there are variables, such as how rigorous the exercise, how tough the opponent and the duration of exercise, that can affect insulin levels, and these variables have to be taken into account in order to get optimal blood sugar control.

Depending on all of these factors, blood insulin levels can fluctuate, causing the blood sugar level to either drop too low, stay within normal range or go higher (as happens in the case in many with poorly controlled diabetes). For the sports-minded person with diabetes—especially the competitive one—the level of blood sugar can be a critical factor in performance. Most athletes with diabetes seem to agree that high blood sugar levels result in less than optimum performance, and that low blood sugar levels may result in poor performance (as well as embarrassment if levels fall so low that a player can begin to feel light-headed and confused, resulting in errors while playing basketball, for instance, that could mean points for the opposition) .

To adequately control diabetes while exercising, an appropriate change in insulin or extra food may be needed. To help determine the necessary adjustments, a home blood sugar test (such as Chemstrip bG, Precision Qid or Accu-chek Advantage) maybe helpful. If it is determined that the blood sugar level is low or normal, extra food before and/or during a period of extended or rigorous exercise is probably wise. The type of food depends on the kind of exercise and when it is performed. For instance, a boxer might consume a form of concentrated sugar with 15 to 30 grams of sugar in it, such as 5 to 10 glucose tablets since he does not want a full stomach. A marathon runner, on the other hand, may consume sugar or liquids and plenty of water or possibly both before and during exercise. In addition, most athletes with diabetes prefer to reduce the amount of insulin taken before a period of extended exercise to reduce the risk of an insulin reaction. For brief periods of exercise, such as sprints or light tennis doubles, no alteration in insulin or food is usually necessary.

How does a doctor know how to adjust a patient's insulin

dose or food intake in order to compensate for a period of exercise? The answer: He doesn't!! As emphasized throughout this book, the person with diabetes must often be his own doctor and estimate how strenuous the exercise will be, how many calories will be burned and whether the insulin injection site is a factor in the rate of insulin absorption. Then, with the help of a sensitive urine test or a self blood sugar test, an appropriate adjustment in insulin or diet can be made if necessary. For very heavy exercise of more than one hour's duration, most athletes prefer to eat less so that they don't exercise on a full stomach. For Type I men this means lowering the insulin dose so that insulin levels don't peak at the height of exercise. For nondiabetics, researchers have shown that insulin is needed but only in very small amounts during exercise. For insulin-dependent people with diabetes in good control, the dose of insulin that is peaking at the height of exercise may be reduced 20% to 70%. In diabetes camps for children where activity and varying strenuous games occur all day long, it is not uncommon to see the insulin dose of the campers reduced by as much as half despite no change in diet.

In my own case, instead of taking my usual pre-breakfast nine units of Regular on a day when I have an early morning tennis match, I may take only four to six units. This is why I like to take insulin four times per day – because it allows me to make an adjustment in insulin if an unanticipated tennis match or sports event comes up. I may not only lower the dose before the event, but even afterward, in addition to eating slightly more after a match as a guard against hypoglycemia. The following table gives a summary guide:

RECOMMENDATIONS FOR UNUSUALLY HEAVY EXERCISE

Control	Keep blood sugar well controlled, with glycohemoglobin less than 10%, preferably under 7%.
Insulin	Drop usual dose that peaks at height of exercise by 20 to 70%.

Food	Same or slightly less, plus eat 10 to 25 grams of simple sugar every 15 to 30 minutes during exercise and extra food afterward.*
Blood sugar tests	Four to seven times per day, including before, during, and after exercise to help determine what level gives you the best performance, and prevent low blood sugar reactions.

* It was reported in the June 1990 issue of *Sports Medicine* that the Ross Laboratory product *Exceed Fluid Replacement and Energy Drink* (available in many supermarkets) does not raise blood sugar as much as simple sugars. It contains a complex glucose polymer that prevents rapid rises in blood sugar and may help to prevent low blood sugar after exercise.

This leads to a key question for the insulin-dependent person: How do you adjust insulin or foods to keep the blood sugar at good levels? The answer to this question varies. For limited exercise such as a 200-meter run or even a mile run, generally no adjustment is needed. However, for heavier exercise some extra calories may be needed. Note the calories burned in the following chart.

Calories Burned Activity Chart

Activity	*Calories Burned per Minute	Per Hour
Thinking, sleeping, resting	1/2-2	40-180
Eating	1/2-2	50-90
Cleaning dishes	1/2-2/5	60-150
Walking, jogging, or running		
1 mile/hour	2-2.5	120-150
2 mile/hour	2.5-4	150-250
Walking, jogging, or running		
3 mile/hour	4-5	250-300
4 mile/hour	6-7	350-420
5 mile/hour	7-9	420-630
6 mile/hour	8-10	480-700
7 mile/hour	10-16	700-1000

Housecleaning, scrubbing	2-6	120-360
Gardening	2-5	150-300
Golf (using cart or walking)	2.5-6	150-300
Tennis (singles or doubles)	2.5-7	150-420
Horseback riding	3-8	180-480
Squash, handball	6-10	420-700
Swimming	5-9	300-630
Cross-country skiing	6-12	420-960
Cycling	3-10	180-700
Dancing (the Twist)	3-8	180-420

*Calories burned are all relative, depending on body weight, air temperature, and the vigor with which one exercises. An easy opponent (most of mine are) will mean less calories burned than a tough one.

It is interesting to note that running four miles may only burn up 400 calories per hour. This means that you can only eat about 400 extra food calories, for example, one sandwich and a glass of Skim milk or possibly a Peter Paul Mounds Bar (preferably the sandwich!). It's also important to realize that the effects of heavy exercise may persist 12 to 24 hours after exercise has stopped, so that hypoglycemia may occur not during exercise but the day after ("the day-after syndrome"). This is most commonly seen when exercise is intermittent and not regular. A cutback in insulin by 10% to 30%, or more food may be needed to prevent hypoglycemia or low blood sugar on the day after exercise. The following are some suggestions:

Practical Pointers for Type I Insulin-Dependent Exercisers

- *Do frequent blood sugar testing* to determine at what level of blood sugar you perform best. One person I know, who compares his method to a jet pilot's, likes to start off the day's activity somewhat high. "I like to start off with my tanks loaded," he says, in order to avoid low blood sugar.

- However, it is now thought that poorly controlled diabetes, where blood sugars are above 200mg% for over a

12-hour period with acetone in the urine, may not only result in a poor performance but may paradoxically raise blood sugars even higher. Most diabetes exercise specialists and athletes with diabetes with whom I have spoken feel that a blood sugar level between 150mg% and 180 mg% prior to the start of heavy exercise is preferable.

- When exercise is intermittently very heavy, *beware of "the day-after syndrome."* The blood sugar-lowering effect of exercise may not be immediate, but when it kicks in, may last up to 24 hours. A friend of mine, a biochemist no less, found this out the hard way. One holiday season he played 3 hours of basketball with his family — much more than he was accustomed to. He had no problem on the day of the exercise, but he passed out the next day from low blood sugar. To avoid this kind of thing from happening, frequent blood sugar testing over at least a 24-hour period after such heavy exercise should be done, and extra food or sugar should always be available.

- *Be careful about very heavy exercise when insulin is peaking.* Insulin may be decreased by 20% to 30% (sometimes more) to prevent the insulin from being too much at the peak of exercise, and, therefore, plenty of sugar will remain in the blood to allow a good performance.

- *Regular exercise is better than intermittent, sporadic exercise.* Regular exercise can result in a significant drop in insulin requirement on a daily basis, sometimes as much as by a third, thus decreasing the chance of low blood sugar.

- *It's crucial to always have some form of sugar available in case it becomes necessary.* Despite your best efforts, low blood sugar can still occur. It's probably wise to consume an equivalent of 1 to 3 teaspoons of sugar every 15 to 30 minutes during prolonged exercise. Here again, *blood sugar testing* will provide the information to decide how many extra calories will be needed.

Exercise for People with Type II Non-Insulin Dependent Diabetes

For the Type II Non-Insulin-Dependent Diabetes, exercise is also helpful in lowering both the blood sugar level and the resistance to insulin that many of them experience. As discussed earlier, non-insulin-dependent people with diabetes have fewer insulin receptors on various body cells (such as muscle, liver, fat or white blood cells), which results in a resistance to insulin.

It has been shown that regular and rigorous exercise can markedly increase the number of functioning receptors, thereby promoting the proper functioning of insulin. This can be true even if the person with diabete does not lose weight (weight loss is another factor that lowers the resistance to the effect of insulin.) When weight loss does occur, as is inevitable with regular exercise, the improvement in diabetes is that much more magnified. Thus, not as much insulin is needed by the pancreas. Non-insulin-dependent people with diabetes should heed the advice of the long-distance runner who, when asked why he ran 1000 miles per year, said, "I'm preserving my pancreas."

Other Effects of Exercise

Besides lowering blood sugar levels, exercise promotes weight reduction by burning more calories and lowering the blood levels of cholesterol and triglycerides. Exercise may also raise levels of HDL cholesterol (high density lipoproteins, the so-called "good cholesterol" that may prevent heart disease), increase longevity by preventing or reducing the severity of heart attacks, and lower blood pressure. In addition, exercise for 30 minutes or more several times per week people feel better both physically and mentally. Although fatigued and depressed prior to exercise, many experience increased strength and heightened spirits during and after exercise. For all of these reasons, *exercise is power.* If possible, it should be treated as an everyday event.

Caution

Despite the many excellent reasons to exercise, some individuals with diabetes should be cautious and should probably obtain their physician's advice before beginning an exercise program. It is important to be sure that heart disease is not present. Some people have heart disease and are not aware of it, because they feel well. For some reason, these people with diabetes may not experience the typical heart symptoms that would alert them to the presence of heart disease. For these patients and for those who know they have heart disease, a good physical examination and a stress electrocardiogram, an exercise heart test, is recommended before beginning an exercise program.

For patients with eye disease, especially proliferative retinopathy, exercise may aggravate their condition. Exercise increases blood pressure during the exercise period and may cause eye bleeding in patients with proliferative retinopathy (see the discussion of retinopathy in Chapter 26, "Complications"). A person with diabetes, even if he has no vision problem, should have an eye check at least once a year to make sure retinopathy is not present.

Exercise with caution if there is circulatory or neuropathy to the legs. If people have impaired circulation, they may not bc able to get enough blood to the exercising muscle, and cramping can occur. Also, these persons should be extremely careful not to get blisters, which could become infected. For the blister-prone person, I would definitely recommend a sock called Double Lay-R (Double Lay-R Sock Co., Doylestown, PA, 215-340-9180). These socks have a thin, two-layer design that cuts down on friction and sweat build-up. The Navy has found them effective in preventing blisters in their field marches, which include carrying a 40-pound pack for 40 to 50 miles. Mountaineers have been particularly impressed. In my own experience, I have found them far superior to anything else I've tried in preventing blisters during my rugged marathon tennis matches (see my tennis story on the following page).

The Doctor at Sport

As you read this section on exercise, you may wonder how this wise doctor/author handles himself when he is exercising. Does he ever get into trouble? As a matter of fact, I did get into trouble. I was initially displaying outstanding athletic skill by building up a 6-0, 3-0 tennis lead against one of my arch rivals. Suddenly, I was overcome by weakness, my legs began to wobble, my tennis strokes fell short, my concentration plummeted, and the score quickly took a turn for the worse to 3-4.

Fortunately, Maureen was nearby and watching the sudden change of events. Realizing that my sugar must have become dangerously low, she offered me a Coke. Thank heaven! Voraciously, I gulped it down. The sugar quickly seeped into my bloodstream and energized me. My tennis opponent, who was temporarily beaming with the thought of a likely comeback, became despondent as my serves smashed in, my speed returned, my volleys became more crisp and accurate, and my concentration became keener. The game was over for my flabbergasted opponent, and I need not tell you the score.

Although this story may exaggerate my tennis ability, it does illustrate the point that it is often difficult to anticipate fluctuations in blood sugar during the throes of exercise. The intensity and duration of the exercise can make all the difference in the world, possibly causing radical shifts in sugar levels. For this reason, quick energy foods should be within easy reach to treat hypoglycemia, should it occur. Don't be embarrassed to carry a carbohydrate with you or to make sure it can be easily obtained. Someone should know you have diabetes, be it your opponent, partner, teammate, or spectator so that he or she can remind you to take sugar in case the mental concentration of a competitive sport makes your medical needs slip your mind. Advise your sport colleagues on hypoglycemic reactions and its varied manifestations!

Exercise does make diabetes easier to control. And since less insulin is needed, the cost of insulin treatment is less. People who exercise feel much better physically and emotionally. As someone who jogs regularly over 900 miles per year and who plays competitive tennis, exercise has helped me achieve good diabetes control. Hopefully, it will continue to help me prevent many of the medical complications caused by diabetes, keeping me healthy and in good shape for those who love and need me.

20

Dental Health and Diabetes

A vital aspect of your daily healthcare regimen is proper dental hygiene. Why? Because cavities can lead to gum disease, which can then result in other serious oral infections that will further complicate your health. As someone with diabetes, you are more prone to the oral infections that can result from dental problems, and are less likely to show signs and symptoms of these infections before they become serious.

Moreover, dental neglect can lead to poor diabetes control (or brittle diabetes). When you don't take good care of your teeth you run the risk of developing health problems that make controlling your diabetes more difficult. And as I've mentioned in Chapter 9, "Insulin— A Miracle Medicine," poor diabetes control seriously affects the overall quality of your life. So, as you can see, preventive dental care for those of us with diabetes is highly important. Fortunately, with a little diligence, you can avoid or at least contain troublesome dental problems. To do so correctly, though, you must understand the connection between dental health and diabetes.

Cavities And Diabetes

Even though the addition of fluoride to water and toothpastes in the early 1960s led to a significant decrease in the incidence of dental caries, cavities are still a fact of life for all of us, but more so for those of us with diabetes. That's because we have higher levels of glucose circulating in our blood. This extra blood sugar spills into the saliva and gingival (gum) fluids, thereby increasing the feeding activity of the bacteria that are already present in the mouth. As the bacteria feed off the extra sugar, they secrete acids that eat away at the protective layer of enamel on our teeth. And it is this process that causes cavities.

Brushing with fluoride toothpastes and using the fluoride rinses that are available both over-the-counter and by prescription will help limit the problem. But regular professional care is really the best way to combat cavities.

Gum Disease And Diabetes

It is estimated that as many as 9 out of 10 otherwise healthy adults have some kind of gum inflammation, which is often the first stage of gum disease. It is also estimated that more than half of all people over 50 have periodontal disease—an advanced form of gum disease.

Dental plaque, the sticky film of bacteria that accumulates daily on tooth surfaces, is the major culprit in gum disease. You may not be able to actually see plaque, but you can usually feel it as a rough, sticky film when you run your tongue along the gumline and across the back of your teeth. Plaque, like dental decay, is also formed by the bacteria that normally inhabit your mouth. These bacteria live off the sugars and starches in the food you eat, and are more active when you consume these kinds of foods. If plaque is not removed promptly and properly, it produces toxic by-products that inflame gum tissue. The irritated gums will slowly pull away from the teeth, creating infected, plaque trapping pockets. As the gums deteriorate further, the bone underneath is exposed to the bacteria. The bone also will begin to deteriorate and cause loose teeth that eventually fall out.

Tartar, or calculus, is another contributor to periodontal disease. It forms when plaque combines with the minerals in your saliva, creating barnacle-like deposits that only professional cleaning can remove.

You are more likely to have these conditions when you let your blood sugar run high, because the extra sugar in your system can overflow into your saliva and gum fluids and, as I described earlier, this process promotes bacterial activity.

When this happens, you will be more likely to accumulate plaque and tartar. If this accumulation is neglected, periodontal disease may set in and may set in earlier and progress faster than it normally would.

Left untreated, a "perio" infection not only causes dental pain and suffering, but also plays havoc with good control of your diabetes. First of all, gum infections can affect your blood sugar levels and thereby your insulin needs. And, if you are on antibiotics to control an infection elsewhere in the body, you may develop a secondary fungal infection in your mouth or develop a resistant strain of mouth bacteria. These infections, in turn, give rise to bad breath or a bad taste or soreness in your mouth. A painful mouth discourages thorough chewing, easily upsetting the strict demands of your diet. Moreover, unchecked gum disease is a leading cause of tooth loss in people with diabetes, which also affects food intake and leads to poor diabetes control.

If you've already lost teeth, you still need to care for the dentures and other dental appliances you may have. Be sure to scrub and soak these appliances regularly in disinfectant solutions (your dental professional can recommend ones to kill the fungi that can creep into the dark, moist crevices of most dental work. Organisms causing infections elsewhere in your body can also set up housekeeping in your dentures. In addition, dentures and bridgework that fit poorly practically guarantee mouth ulcers. These ulcers provide a site of broken skin that invites further infection and pain. This makes proper chewing difficult, and affects your ability to follow your diabetes diet.

What You Can Do

There are a number of simple measures you can take to preserve your teeth and maintain healthy gums. The most important first step you can take is to strictly control your blood glucose levels. Other important ways to prevent problems include: good home oral hygiene, regular checkups, effective plaque removal and prompt treatment if necessary.

Home Care

Practice good oral hygiene at home every day. This simply means that you should brush with a soft-bristle toothbrush (they are less abrasive to your gums) and floss regularly. Make sure that you let your toothbrush dry thoroughly between uses. In other words don't keep it in a dark, damp place because this allows the growth of bacteria that can infect your mouth. Also, it is best to replace your toothbrush every three months. Electric toothbrushes and irrigators can be used, if you prefer, to clean hard-to-reach spaces between teeth where plaque readily accumulates; these instruments are especially helpful for patients with vision or manual dexterity problems. However, avoid over-brushing or brushing too vigorously with these devices, since they can abrade gums, exposing sensitive tooth roots. If you are uncertain about how to brush and floss properly, ask your dentist or the dental hygienist to show you the right technique.

Check-Ups

You should have a thorough dental exam at least twice a year. However, if your gums bleed when you eat or brush your teeth or if you notice any other unusual changes in your mouth, such as patches of whitish-colored skin (an indication of oral cancer), see a dentist immediately.

People with Type I diabetes should closely follow medication guidelines to make sure no high or low sugar reactions occur during the exam or, more importantly, during a dental procedure. The morning is generally the best time for most insulin-dependent patients to schedule checkups and treatments.

When you have an appointment, report your most recent blood sugar reading. Also, he honest about how well—or poorly—you've controlled your diabetes. Your dentist may want to confirm control with a spot check. And, be sure to communicate any fears or concerns about the procedure you're about to undergo so that the dentist can put your mind at ease. Dental fear can cause you undue stress that will affect your insulin needs.

Diet and insulin are important before, during, and after a procedure. If you anticipate that a dental procedure will make chewing difficult while you are recovering, have your dentist and diabetes specialist talk to each other beforehand to determine your post-procedure dietary and insulin needs.

It is also important to complete the required medical history form as accurately as possible so that the dental staff will be aware of your individual insulin needs and can modify your dental treatment, if necessary. Your dentist will probably ask you additional questions related to your condition, such as how long have you had your diabetes, what type it is, medications you are on, how often you have a reaction (such as a hypoglycemic or ketoacidic reaction), when you last visited the dentist and the time since your last meal. Be sure to volunteer this information if you aren't asked.

You can have normal-looking gums, yet have an infection lurking beneath them. Therefore, a complete periodontal exam will include: an evaluation of the gums for any signs of inflammation; analysis for plaque; testing for perio pockets, bone loss and tooth mobility; and application of gum pressure around each and every tooth to check for puss or any discharge. Now a days, testing for periodontal disease includes a series of laboratory analysis in addition to the visual signs your dentist will look for during your visit, so you can ask your dentist about the need to have such an analysis done. Your evaluation should also include an examination for oral lesions or cancer, and for such conditions as dry mouth, lupus, scleroderma, and jaw arthritis. In addition, any dental devices you may have should be evaluated for proper fit to avoid the mouth ulcers I mentioned earlier in this chapter.

Plaque Removal

Once the presence of plaque has been established, your dentist, hygienist, or periodontist (a dental specialist in periodontal disease) will use special instruments to probe periodontal pockets and scrape toothroot surfaces in order to remove all plaque and tartar. Surgical repositioning of gum tissue to eliminate pockets around teeth may also be required. In addition to these mechanical methods of plaque control, there are also a number of antibacterial approaches to treatment. They range from "degerming" baths to antibiotic treatments and rinses. You'll also receive nutritional (such as vitamin and mineral intake) recommendations. Mild cases of plaque build-up will need treatment once every few months; more serious cases may require weekly treatments.

Treatment

If you have an advanced stage of gum disease, you may need the specialized care of a periodontist, a dentist who specializes in periodontal disease and is therefore well-equipped to handle the more complex treatments that gum problems require. If a tooth requires root-canal therapy, an endodontist, a specialist in dental nerve treatment, would be involved.

Before any procedure, be sure to ask the dentist how complex the procedure will be and whether you will be able to eat normally afterwards. Then consult your doctor or diabetes specialist about any needed adjustments in your diet or in your insulin requirements so that you can avoid low or high blood sugar reactions. Your insulin levels may need modification before, as well as after, a visit. It is therefore a good idea to bring your glucose testing device with you so that on-the-spot checks of your blood sugar level can be done as the procedure is carried out. If gum surgery is required, make sure you have your diabetes well under control; otherwise, healing may take longer.

When undergoing any extended treatment, don't try to be a hero or heroine when it comes to the pain or discomfort from a dental procedure. Otherwise, the stress of the pain can influence your sugar levels and alter your normal insulin needs. Your dentists and the dental staff can suggest stress and anxiety-reducing methods ahead of time, which you can begin practicing well before your dental work is scheduled.

Discuss ways to limit discomfort as well. Most of all, reassure yourself that the dental professionals who are treating you are knowledgeable about what to do in the event of an emergency, so put any undue fears to rest.

Your dental caregivers are important members of your health-care team. So, you can expect them to work closely with your doctor to ensure consistency in your overall treatment. They will make sure that your special needs are met to successfully complete the dental procedure you may need.

So, as you can see, as long as you follow the basic principles of prevention, including a regimen of daily oral hygiene, regular dental check-ups and proper treatment as needed, you are certain to minimize your dental problems—and good teeth certainly mean good health.

21

Care of the Skin

"She is known by the beauty of her skin..."   Unknown Author

According to a survey by *Diabetes Self Management Magazine*, 87% of people with diabetes polled use some kind of hand and body cream, lotion or oil. I would guess that a majority of those who responded to the survey were women, since it is usually my female patients who express anxiety over the effects diabetes may be having on their skin, and it is usually these patients who make sure their skin looks good. These women are rightfully concerned about the health and appearance of their skin. However, it is a concern that must be shared among women and men, alike, because the skin of both can be affected by diabetes.

Skin and its Functions

Why should both men and women take care of their skin? Because the skin does more than simply contribute to one's appearance. The skin protects the body from excess cold, heat, wind and sun to prevent dehydration, and is the first line of defense against infections. To fulfill its many roles, the skin has to be healthy. It needs adequate nutrition to maintain its strength and tone in order to resist injuries from minor trauma. And it needs adequate moisture to prevent cracking, peeling or fissuring—all of which can cause breaks in the skin through which infectious agents can enter.

Effects of Diabetes on Skin

As I mentioned in Chapter 4, "Subtle Signs of Diabetes," changes in the skin are often the initial signs of diabetes. More specifically, the skin can show signs of poor diabetes control. These "signs" include boils or skin abscesses, which actually result from bacterial infections. Fungal infections can also develop, which show up as breaks in the skin, redness, itching or malador. The reason that people with diabetes are more prone to these types of skin infections is because of the increased amounts of glucose in the skin, and certain organisms such as *Candida* and *Monila* yeasts thrive in a high-sugar environment. Extra blood glucose is often stored in the skin, and this glucose attracts the organisms that normally live on the skin or in the surrounding atmosphere (especially around the sweaty, moist areas of the body, such as feet, genitals and underneath breasts). Prolonged cases of uncontrolled diabetes can lead to more serious skin infections because high blood sugar affects the ability of white blood cells (which are part of the body's immune system) to kill bacteria.

Moreover, poor control accelerates the development of such problems as diabetes neuropathy, a complication that affects the nervous system. When the nervous system is affected, the sweat and sebaceous glands in the skin don't work correctly to prevent excessive water loss. The blood vessels that supply the skin may also be affected, impairing the delivery of water and nutrients via blood to the skin. On top of that, when diabetes control is poor, there may be nerve damage to the extent that a wound does not cause any pain. Consequently, the wound may go unnoticed and left open and untreated, putting the patient at risk for an infection.

People with diabetes commonly develop dry skin (which can cause the skin and nails to become thickened) and may suffer some hair loss. Dry skin is a particularly troublesome problem for many individuals with diabetes. High blood sugar (over 180mg%) can occur without any outwardly noticeable symptoms, yet can lead to internal problems such as excessive loss of water from the skin and body through increased urination. Thus, the skin is left dehydrated, and if left untreated, can develop cracks or fissures that, as I've mentioned, lead to various skin infections.

Other possible skin problems include pruritus (itching);

yellowish or brown lesions that develop when diabetes is uncontrolled (they disappear when the diabetes is brought under control); and shin spots, brownish patches about the size of a dime that are thought to occur after incidental bumps to the shins.

Daily Skin Care: Hydrate and Lubricate

Since dry skin is the most common skin problem that people with diabetes face, keeping the skin moist and supple is by far the most important step in daily care. Basically, dry skin is caused by the loss of water from the outer skin layer as well as lack of sufficient supply of nutrients in the skin tissue such as vitamins and essential fatty acids. However, the elasticity and texture of healthy skin also depends on the presence of hydrophilic lipids (fats that absorb water) in the outer part of the skin. Other general causes of dry skin include hot, dry weather, dehumidifiers in the home, saunas, and cosmetics and skin care preparations containing alcohol (which remove water from the uppermost layer of the skin). These factors can exacerbate an existing dry skin problem in people with diabetes. Therefore, it is important to take the proper steps in preventing dry skin by preserving or supplementing the water and lipid content of the skin, and to carefully consider the kind of products—lotions, creams, oils or cosmetics that you use.

General Care Guidelines

Daily care of the skin is vital to overall health—for both men and women. The following guidelines should become part of your everyday health and skin care regimen:
• Don't let diabetes become or stay out of control. Work with your health care team to maintain tight control of your blood sugar levels. Maintaining stable levels will prevent the skin infections that can occur when excess glucose is stored in the skin, and the other complications that result from high blood sugar levels. Controlling your diet is, of

course, paramount in keeping blood sugar levels in check. Eat a nutritious diet that includes fresh fruits and vegetables and adequate amounts of vitamins A, B$_6$, C, D and E, and monounsaturated fats such as olive oil. Also drink 6 to 8 glasses of water daily.

- Check the general condition of your skin with your doctor regularly; make an appointment as soon as you notice a change in coloration or any lesion that is not normal.
- Bathe or shower in lukewarm water rather than hot water to reduce the amount of water evaporation from the skin's surface. Cleanse with a mild soap or gel, and avoid deodorant soaps which strip surface oils and can irritate skin. Products such as Neutrogena or Aveeno cleansers are generally recommended because they clean without excessively drying out the skin. Use a gentle cleanser with moisturizing qualities such as ANASTASIA MARIE® Diabetic Pure Skin Therapy® *Purifying Cleansing Lotion* by Anastasia Marie Laboratories, Inc. (1-800-542-7546), which is extremely mild yet effective in removing impurities without stripping the skin of its natural oils.
- Apply a moisturizing cream or lotion immediately after a bath or shower. This will preserve adequate moisture in your skin, preventing the cracking, peeling and fissuring that can often lead to infections. A penetrating body oil used during and after bathing will replenish oils and seal in moisture. Your physician can recommend products that are appropriate for you.
- Apply creams or lotions with sunscreen of SPF 15 or more to all exposed areas to protect against damage and skin irritation from sun and ultraviolet rays.
- For extra-dry skin, lubricating moisturizing creams can be applied to the skin.
- When caring for your skin, don't forget to care for your feet as well. Moisturize and inspect your feet daily to prevent dry, rough and scaly skin. Apply lubricating moisturizing creams to soothe cracked heels, calluses and chapped skin.

   This last point is particularly important. People with diabetes will develop foot complications during the course of their diabetes. These complications can include brittle toe-nails, sores and infections, numbness in the toes and feet and nighttime leg cramps. It is essential, therefore, to pay special attention to your feet, and to take regular care of the skin in this area. The following chapter (Foot Care) will detail the special foot problems that can occur in individuals with dia-betes, and provide information on how to care for the skin on your feet.

It has been my experience that skin and foot care products made by Anastasia Marie Laboratories, Inc. (1-800-542-7546) can help many of the problems I have mentioned. Anastasia Shehak is a registered dietician, a licensed dietician, and a certified diabetes educator and has had diabetes for over 28 years. She developed a line of products, ANASTASIA MARIE® Diabetic Pure Skin Therapy®, after a long and fruit-less search for the best skin care products for people with diabetes. Since she found none of the commercially available products satisfactory, Anastasia, R.D., L.D., CDE, with the help of a team of medical physicians, endocrinologists, dermatologists, podiatrists, and pharmacists developed products specifically formulated for people with diabetes. They are made of natural ingredients, vitamins, antioxidants, and plant extracts, without alcohol or petroleum products which tend to dry and irritate the skin. Her line of products are formulated for both men and women. In fact, I've been using ANASTASIA MARIE® Diabetic Pure Skin Therapy® products by Anastasia Marie Laboratories, Inc. for several years and am quite happy with the results.

Before choosing any skin care product, though, it is best o consult with your physician. Since each person has very individual skin care needs, your physician can recommend products appropriate for your use.

22

Foot Care

Foot problems can occur during the course of diabetes. These complications include dry, brittle toenails, pain, tingling, or numbness of the toes and feet, sores on the toes and the soles of the feet; foot inflammations and infections, and night cramps in the legs. The most dreaded complication, gangrene, can be avoided with special attention to general foot hygiene. The two main foot problems are neuropathy and poor circulation.

As discussed earlier, *neuropathy* can cause a lessening or complete loss of sensation. For example, if you were to step on a sharp object such as a tack and not experience pain, you may very well have diabetes neuropathy. There are varying degrees of loss of feeling. You may be aware of excruciating pain (as in gout or severe injury) but not of minor injuries such as stubbing your toe. You may not feel pain at the time but later notice a cut or bruise. The exact cause of diabetes neuropathy is not completely understood, but there seems to be some connection between the severity of diabetes neuropathy and prolonged periods of excessively high blood sugar levels.

Poor circulation, most common in people who have had diabetes for a long period of time, also contributes to foot problems. Circulation usually deteriorates with age, even in people who do not have diabetes.

As discussed in Chapter 26, "Complications," diabetes can affect the small arterial vessels. Since those vessels in the feet are farthest from the heart, they become the prime targets for poor circulation. These blood vessels age more rapidly than normal and become clogged so that they are no longer able to transport enough blood to the feet. Since a sufficient blood supply is necessary for normal maintenance of body tissues, the feet and legs are the first to become adversely affected when circulation is inadequate. An early indication of this condition is a cramp-like pain experienced when walking a moderate distance. Another early sign is poor healing of any abrasion or open cut. If a person with diabetes feet look red when sitting, this is a later indication of poor circulation. It is important to pay attention to these signs and consult a doctor if any of them are present.

On a general note, if you are a person with diabetes, whether or not you use insulin, you should inform the doctors that treat you (including your podiatrist and dentist) that you have diabetes.

Daily Foot Care

To maintain proper foot care and avoid problems with your feet, it is necessary to perform a daily routine of general foot care, hygiene, and inspection.

You should wash your feet daily with warm water, not hot water. Check the water temperature with your hand. Hot water can burn and damage the skin on your feet, and if you have neuropathy, you may not be aware of any damage. When taking a foot bath, use only a mild, nonmedicated soap. If you prefer, a tub bath can suffice. After bathing, dry the feet carefully. Make sure to dry thoroughly between the toes, without pulling the towel vigorously between them, to help prevent fungal infections.

Feet Examination

Once your feet are clean and dry, examine them very closely in adequate light. If your eyesight is poor, have someone inspect your feet for you. Look for blisters, cuts, or scratches. Any break in the skin is a potential area of infection and should be treated at home with great care.

If you find a skin break or blister, apply a mild antiseptic such as isopropyl alcohol, Bactine, ST-37, Merthiolate, or Metaphen to the area. Then cover the area with a dry, sterile dressing and secure in place with nonallergenic tape such as Micro Pore or any other paper tape. Do not apply adhesive tape, muleskin, or other occlusive dressing directly over the infected area. Iodine preparations, carbolic acid, and creosol should never be used. Also, do not use commercial preparations such as Lysol, epsom salts, or boric acid in foot soaks unless prescribed by your physician or podiatrist.

Never use hot water bottles or heating pads of any kind on your feet. At the first sign of pain, redness, or swelling, consult your physician or podiatrist.

Lubrication

After washing, drying, and inspecting the feet, apply a blended lubricating cream to your feet to prevent dryness and cracks in the skin. There are various commercial preparations available (Eucerin, Nivea, Dermassage, and Alpha-Keri Lotion to name a few). As I mentioned in the previous chapter, ANASTASIA MARIE® Diabetic Pure Skin Therapy® (1-800-542-7546) products are my favorite. Avoid the areas around the toenails and in between the toes unless you are using ANASTASIA MARIE® Diapedic Foot Cream and Diapedic® Foot Oil. Her foot cream is the only one that can be used between the toes as it contains antifungal and anti-bacterial agents.

Care of Toenails

Cut nails short in the center and never below the juncture of the nail and the flesh at the corners. Never dig into the corners of the nails. File your toenails with a diamond-type file, and never file shorter than the end of the toe. If your toenails are thick, discolored, hard, and tend to split when being filed, have your podiatrist trim them for you. Sometimes when toenails have become thickened, it's because of a fungus infection. Ask your doctor about a topical treatment called Loprox, and also how the toenails can be filed down to help limit the infection.

Care of Corns and Calluses

Never cut corns or calluses since you do not have the proper tools or the skill and cannot achieve the proper position to do so. Chemical agents such as corn cures should also be avoided. Salicylic acid preparations destroy tissue without causing pain, and they are very dangerous.

Footwear

Never walk barefoot inside or outside the house. Shoes offer more protection than slippers, but slippers with sturdy toes can be worn around the house to prevent injury from toe stubbing.

Since any object that creates pressure or a break in the skin may cause irritation or infection, you should inspect the insides of your shoes for foreign objects, nail points, and torn linings. Avoiding wet feet, wet shoes, or wet socks, especially in the winter months, should also help prevent foot infection.

Shoes and Slippers

It is very important to select your shoes carefully, making sure they fit properly, providing enough room for all the toes to be in their natural positions, and allowing for toe motion. New shoes should be broken in gradually to prevent blister formation. Avoid wearing shoes with pointed toes, since they prevent proper foot position. Open-toe or open-heel shoes should also be avoided, since they do not provide enough protection for your feet.

Socks

Make sure to wear machine-washable cotton or wool socks with your shoes and to change your socks daily to ensure cleanliness. Avoid mended socks as well as socks with seams or constricting tops. Circular garters or any other support garment that causes local constriction should not be worn since they prevent proper blood circulation.

Socks should always be large enough to allow considerable toe motion. If the toes overlap or are too close together, separate them with lamb's wool.

Finally, as I mention in the chapter on exercise, Double Lay-R socks are comfortable and provide excellent absorption and protection from blisters. I would recommend them for everyday use as well as for athletics.

Final Tips

Final tips related to general foot care are:

- Do not smoke. The nicotine in tobacco shrinks the blood vessels and slows down blood flow to the feet.
- Avoid extreme temperatures. Keep your feet at or above room temperature as much or the time as possible.
- Exercise. Walking improves circulation and is the best exercise for your feet.
- Avoid blisters. To avoid blisters, be careful with new footwear, especially if they're tight or pointy. For anyone who's prone to getting blisters, especially if neuropathy is present, consider wearing special socks. And don't forget Double Lay-R socks (Double Lay R Sock Co., 62 West State Street, Doylestown, PA; 215-340-9180) which are particularly helpful in preventing blisters.
- For any lesion or opening on foot with drainage, or if there is redness or swelling, it is important to be evaluated by a physician immediately for possible antibiotic treatment.
- Use a lubricating moisturizing foot cream or oil (such as ANASTASIA MARIE® Diabetic Pure Skin Therapy™, Diapedic® Foot Cream and Diapedic® Foot Oil; 1-800-542-7546) twice a day to help prevent dryness.

23

Women and Diabetes: Menses, Sexual Response and Pregnancy

Menses

The menses, commonly called the "period," or menstruation, refers to the vaginal bleeding that occurs in women every 28 to 36 days. In some women, the interval can be less than 28 days or more than 36 days and still be normal. This bleeding results from the sloughing off of the cells that line the uterus.

These uterine cells, triggered by the female hormones estrogen and progesterone (produced by the ovaries), accumulate in order to nourish the egg that has become embedded in the uterine lining as it awaits fertilization. When fertilization does not occur, the concentration of estrogen and progesterone become very low and cease to stimulate the growth of the cells. Bleeding results over the next 3 to 5 days until the estrogen concentration again starts to increase during the next menstrual cycle. Associated with menstruation and the related hormonal changes are several symptoms that include swelling of the hands and feet, cramps, nausea, and irritability.

The menarche, or the age when menstruation first begins, usually occurs between 12 and 14 years of age. When a woman has diabetes, the menarche may be somewhat delayed. This is particularly true when the diabetes has been poorly controlled as a result of insufficient insulin, overeating, or poor nutrition. This causes a disturbance in the usual hormonal balance, which results in impaired physical development. Once the female with diabetes properly adjusts her insulin dose and adopts a more nutritionally balanced diet, the menarche should occur. If the menarche does not then

177

occur, other medical possibilities should be explored to explain the condition. Sometimes it is normal for the menarche to start as late as 16 years of age, particularly if this is a family trait.

Poorly controlled diabetes can also affect the regularity of the cycle. It is uncertain whether mental stress, hormonal imbalance, poor nutrition, or other factors associated with poor control cause menstrual irregularity. In any case, good diabetes control usually means a more regular cycle.

Just as diabetes can affect menstruation, menstruation and the associated hormonal changes, in turn, can possibly affect diabetes. Women with diabetes can easily manage and anticipate these effects with a little knowledge.

For example, as the levels of estrogen and progesterone increase just prior to menstruation, there is some resistance to insulin, which can lead to elevated blood sugar levels. Type I insulin-dependent women may, therefore, need to make a slight adjustment in insulin (higher dose) or reduce their food intake in order to counteract this tendency toward higher blood sugar. For the Type II non-insulin-dependent woman, reduced food intake is also appropriate just prior to menstruation. Once the menstrual cycle begins, estrogen and progesterone production decrease and blood sugar levels tend to fall as well (nausea often accompanies this drop in blood sugar; women can use this as a possible sign of decreasing sugar). For those using insulin, a smaller dose during menstruation may help prevent this tendency.

Menopause

The menopause, commonly referred to as the "change of life," is the point at which menstruation stops, usually sometime after age 40. At menopause, various changes start to take place. Ovulation ceases, and there is marked by a reduction in estrogen and progesterone production. Accompanying these changes are a number of unpleasant symptoms including depression, headache, hot flashes, and as the woman gets older, a tendency toward brittleness of bones and resulting fractures. These symptoms occur in varying degrees with different women, and some women barely experience any of them at all.

"Hot flashes" can be one of the more disturbing and potentially embarrassing symptoms of menopause. The term refers to the sudden onset of the sensation of heat waves passing through the body accompanied by excessive perspiration, weakness and headache. These hot flashes can occur once a day or more than 10 times a day.

For the woman with diabetes, hot flashes can be even more exasperating as the symptoms may be confused with hypoglycemia, which cause similar reactions. This confusion can greatly complicate proper diabetes control. For instance, if a woman mistakes her hot flashes for hypoglycemia, she may take extra sugar or food, elevating blood sugar levels. Conversely, if she mistakes her hypoglycemia symptoms for hot flashes, she may fail to take sugar and her low blood sugar reaction will become even more severe. Fortunately, there are ways to avoid confusion. By testing urine with a sensitive urine test or, even better, by testing her own blood sugar with one of the self blood sugar methods that are now available, a woman should be able to tell whether her symptoms are due to hypoglycemia or menopause.

Depression can also occur during and after menopause. A full discussion of depression is beyond the scope of this book, but it is thought to be partially related to the reduced estrogen concentration that occurs during menopause. For the woman with diabetes, mental stress, overeating, or undereating (often associated with depression), and use of any antidepressive medication can affect blood sugar metabolism and proper diabetes control.

Brittleness of bones (osteoporosis) that can occur in varying degrees during or after menopause can lead to bone weakness and even fractures. Since diabetes itself can lead to bone brittleness, menopause in the woman with diabetes often compounds the problem, and exercise may have to be restricted.

There is some evidence that brittle bones may be

prevented by a diet high in calcium (at least 800mg per day) and adequate in vitamin D (400 IU). If a patient's diet does not allow for one quart of milk per day (which contains the above supply of calcium and vitamin D) or sufficient amounts of other foods high in these nutrients, an ample amount of calcium can be easily and cheaply obtained from two Tums per day. Vitamin D supplement should be added, however.

Given the above discussion on menopause, is there anything that can be done to alleviate these unpleasant symptoms? Since the symptoms seem to be a manifestation of reduced estrogen production by the ovaries, supplemental intake of estrogen should be considered. After menopause, estrogen replacement is definitely important. It can prevent many of the effects of hormone deficiency. It can prevent osteoporosis, protect against heart disease, have a beneficial effect on the cholesterol, on the skin and vaginal surfaces, and improve the mood. However, there is controversy about the use of estrogen, since some medical studies indicate that estrogen supplementation may he associated with a slight in crease in the incidence of cancer of the uterus and possible other medical problems. The use of estrogen is thus a complicated issue, and women with particularly severe menopausal symptoms should consult their doctor. There are two more medications that may also prevent osteoporosis: Calcimal, an injection and Fosamax. Both medications may be helpful against bone loss and help rebuild bone.

Sexual Response

Sexual response in a woman involves a desire for intimacy, followed by sexual arousal, and finally resolution through orgasm. The biological processes that elicit the response are complex, involving not only psychological factors, but also the endocrine, vascular and neurological systems. If any of these systems go awry, the intensity of the sexual response may be affected, resulting in a marked decrease.

For example, a common neurological problem many

people with diabetes face is diabetes neuropathy, a degenerative nerve disease that generally occurs in people with diabetes who have had poor control of their blood glucose levels over a period of several years. If significant neuropathy occurs in a woman with diabetes, the pleasurable sensation that results from the stimulation of the genitalia, particularly the clitoris, may be impaired and the rhythmic contractions that occur during climax may not be as satisfying. Other neurological responses, such as swelling and lubrication of the vagina and swelling of the nipples, may also be affected.

Poor diabetes control can also disturb the normal circulation of a woman's hormones. Just as poor control results in a hormonal imbalance that affects a woman's menstrual cycle, so can it influence the level of hormones that regulate a woman's libido. In addition, the lower hormonal levels will lead to inadequate vaginal lubrication, resulting in pain and discomfort during intercourse.

Moreover, the constantly fluctuating and insufficient blood sugar levels that result from poor control can leave a woman feeling tired, lifeless and depressed. Consequently, she may lose her desire for sex. Poor diabetes control can also lead to an irritating vaginal yeast infection or unpleasant vaginal discharges, which can lessen a woman's enjoyment with intercourse. Thus, a low state of arousal (caused by neurological or hormonal problems) and the physical discomfort (from a vaginal infection) can make it more difficult for a woman with diabetes to experience an orgasm, further inhibiting her interest in sex. When any of these problems occur, a woman may simply avoid intercourse—much to the dismay of her partner.

However, before we attribute these problems solely to poor diabetes control, keep in mind that problems such as decreased vaginal lubrication and the resultant pain and irritation during intercourse can also be caused by the decreased hormone levels that accompany the onset of menopause. So, women in their late forties and fifties should consider menopause as a cause of any of the problems I've just described. All women experiencing these symptoms can discuss therapeutic options, such as hormonal replacement therapy and vaginal lubricants, with her physician.

Diabetes does not have to prevent a woman's enjoyment of intimacy. The problems that I've just described can be avoided or eliminated quite simply with good blood sugar control. Keeping track of blood sugar levels and maintaining as tight control as possible can overcome the two common hurdles that a woman with diabetes can face.

By keeping in good health with nutritional supplements, diet and exercise, a woman can enjoy normal levels of arousal. Basically, an otherwise healthy woman with diabetes— one who is in good physical shape with her blood sugar levels firmly under control—should experience as much satisfaction in her sexual love relationship as any other woman without diabetes.

Pregnancy

Among physicians, there is almost universal agreement that the closer to normal that blood sugars are maintained during pregnancy, the better the outcome. Even for the mother without diabetes, pregnancy is not easy because of discomfort, weight gain and a tendency for problems such as varicose veins and bladder infections. But for the woman with diabetes, pregnancy also means paying very strict attention to diet, regulating insulin intake (if insulin is needed) and, in some cases, sharply limiting her activities.

Thanks to present-day medical management, women with can experience a successful pregnancy. Twenty years ago, however, this was not the case. Babies of women with diabetes have been faced with a high risk of mortality. The improvement that has occurred over the past few decades as have results from improved diabetes control and better methods of determining when delivery should occur.

Pregnancy causes dramatic changes in a woman's body. One effect is a marked change in a woman's hormonal out-put, which usually occurs after the third month. As a result, sugar is not utilized as efficiently. In addition, the placenta produces hormones that block the effect of insulin. These hormonal changes sometimes trigger the development of diabetes in a previously woman without diabetes. This condition is called gestational or pregnancy diabetes. Generally, experts feel that this condition develops if the rising or fasting blood sugar exceeds 105mg% or the after-eating blood sugar exceeds 120mg%. For the majority of women, the diabetes will disappear once pregnancy is over, but for others, the diabetes may be permanent.

For the woman who has diabetes prior to pregnancy, the changes associated with pregnancy lead to increased difficulty in controlling the diabetes. In the early stages of pregnancy, morning sickness may occur, possibly because of decreased food intake. At the same time, the uterus and developing baby may be using more calories! As a result, it is possible that the woman with diabetes may need less insulin during the first 2 to 3 months of pregnancy. It is very important to monitor both the caloric and insulin intake during this period to avoid the risk of insulin reactions.

As pregnancy continues, hormones are produced that block the effect of insulin and create a tendency toward high blood sugar. As a result, it is common to need more than twice as much insulin later in pregnancy in order to get blood sugars in the near-normal range and to keep it there. High blood sugar strains the fetal pancreas and may produce high blood insulin levels in the fetus. These factors may result in "big babies" or create respiratory problems and other complications, including hypoglycemia, in the newborn.

It is clear that maintaining normal blood sugars is the way to ensure the best possible outcome of the pregnancy. How is this accomplished? By controlling blood sugars through diet or through both diet and insulin. With the aid of frequent blood sugar and urine tests, normal blood sugar levels can be maintained. Diet alone may be satisfactory for those who had mild diabetes before pregnancy or those with pregnancy diabetes. However, diet control alone has some drawbacks. Current medical thinking stresses that during pregnancy, a fairly large number of calories is necessary to assure adequate nutrition for the infant. An average of 1700 to 2500 calories per day (from foods relatively high in calcium, protein, and carbohydrate) is recommended. The diet cannot be greatly restricted in an attempt to control the blood sugar, as it might be in the nonpregnant woman. Even the overweight woman who might otherwise go on a restricted diet must postpone such a diet until after pregnancy to avoid the potential hazards to the baby caused by undernutrition. A weight gain of 25 to 30 pounds during the course of pregnancy is now considered healthiest for the mother and baby.

It is important that the woman understand all aspects of any diet and that she measure her food intake rather than "guesstimate" it, since estimated totals can be off by as much as 500 calories. Several visits with a diet counselor may be necessary in order to arrive at the proper diet, which should be between 1700 to 2500 calories. This diet may result in elevated blood sugar. Most experts feel that the fasting blood sugar that occurs in the morning when a woman first wakes up should be less than 100mg%, and the after-meal blood sugar between 90mg% and 120mg%. For gestational diabetes blood sugars that are exceeding the limits, insulin will be needed, according to most experts. In cases where a woman is introduced to insulin for the first time, it may be appropriate for her to be hospitalized for complete instructions concerning insulin use, especially when the blood sugars are far above these limits, so that they can rapidly be brought down. In the hospital she can be given thorough instructions and supervision on the use of insulin as needed for good control.

The Type I insulin-dependent woman will need the same type of diet as that prescribed for a woman whose diabetes who can be controlled with diet alone. If blood sugars become elevated, more insulin will be needed.

To monitor the effects of diet and insulin on the control of diabetes, blood sugar tests are necessary. "Fasting" blood sugar and "after-eating" (postprandial) blood sugar tests should be taken anywhere between 2 to 10 times per day, depending on the degree of control. If control is not good, more frequent blood sugar determinations may be necessary. Blood sugars should be ideally kept between 60mg% and 90mg% before meals and under 120mg% after meals. If we assume that the mother is on the right diet, any elevation above these levels may be an indication that more insulin is needed. Any change in therapy of a pregnant woman should be made under the supervision of the physician (family physician, diabetes specialist, or obstetrician) taking primary responsibility for control of the diabetes.

While urine sugar tests are not especially helpful in monitoring insulin therapy, testing for urine ketones (acetone) is useful. Ketonuria can result from undereating ("starvation ketosis") or from lack of insulin and poor diabetes control. Either condition is potentially harmful, and an appropriate change in therapy is indicated: either more food or more insulin (the latter if the patient is following the appropriate diet and is not overeating).

It is important to monitor the general health of the pregnant woman as well as her blood sugar and urine acetone. This will mean fairly frequent visits to the doctor to measure blood pressure, to examine the eyes for retinopathy and to check for other problems such as bladder infections. All of these problems could be present without obvious symptoms, and routine examination can lead to early detection of any complications. If any problems are present, they should be treated at once.

The previous discussion has dealt primarily with keeping the mother in good health. Another important issue is determining the best time for the delivery of the baby. In the past, before diabetes could be controlled, there was a moderate chance that the baby would not survive a full term pregnancy. Because of this, it was common to deliver the baby by Caesarean section early sometime between the 33rd and the 37th week. Sometimes this was too early and the baby was not mature or strong enough to resist disease. One frequent consequence of such an early delivery was respiratory distress syndrome (also known as hyaline membrane disease), where the newborn's lungs lack surfactant, a soapy substance that lends to the elasticity of the lungs.

Today, however, with the much improved methods of monitoring fetal progress, pregnancies can be prolonged in almost all cases until the baby is strong enough for delivery. These methods include measuring the fetus heart rate in response to contractions of the uterus, measuring estrogen levels of the woman (which are usually very high in pregnancy) and using amniocentesis to measure the levels of lecithin and sphingomyelin (fats produced by the fetal lungs) in the fluid inside the uterus. The latter helps determine whether the fetal lungs will be mature enough to accept the job of breathing at birth.

These tests are usually done from the 32nd to 34th week on, at weekly, or bi-weekly intervals depending on how well the pregnancy is proceeding. Using their results, the physician will choose the best time and method of delivery.

By using the monitoring techniques that are currently available and by availing herself of proper medical care, the woman with diabetes can expect to give birth to a healthy baby. It does require her dedication, as implied by the foregoing discussion, and in many instances, some financial burden. But the reward of a healthy newborn makes any personal or financial commitment tremendously worthwhile.

Control of Diabetes After Pregnancy

After the pregnancy, women who had developed gestational diabetes may find blood sugars returning to normal. Good diet, exercise, and blood sugar checks are important in minimizing the potential for the diabetes to redevelop. For some women with gestational diabetes, the diabetes will persist and efforts to control it should therefore continue. For these women, as well as for the woman who had diabetes before pregnancy, the insulin requirements will become markedly reduced just after childbirth—so much so that very little is needed for the first few days following delivery. So, care must be taken to avoid insulin reactions. Gradually, the insulin requirements will return to pre-pregnancy levels. After a successful pregnancy with her concerns relieved, it is natural for a woman to relax and diabetes control tends to loosen up a bit. However, as the baby grows, a routine develops, and this reinforces the mother's efforts toward good control.

Pam "Has Her Second Baby"

Pam was only 22 years old, yet she was plagued by medical problems since the tender age of 6 years, that she never dreamed could happen to her. Her diabetes was never well controlled for a number of reasons, we know all too well: the irregular eating habits of a very young girl, the rebellious eating habits of an impressionable adolescent desiring to be like her peers, ignorance of healthy eating habits and the proper use of insulin, lack of education about her disease, lack of knowledge for the prevention of illness and disease and finally, lack of motivation lead to repeated. This lack of control lead to repeated hospitalization, the developement of hypertension, requiring five different blood pressure medicines and renal failure. By the time Pam came to me, as a patient, she had spent six months of that year in and out of the hospital and sadly, this forced her to postpone her anticipated marriage to Christopher.

Her doctor was chagrined, attributing her problems to psychological reasons, rebellion and non-compliance.

Yet, I saw something in Pam, that touched me and told me, she sincerely wanted a better life for herself. It was also obvious she had real medical problems, that needed prompt attention.

This is what happened. Pam was seen immediately by a kidney specialist, who realized that her high blood pressure requiring so many medications, was caused by kidney disease. He recommended a kidney transplant.

With Chritopher and her family at her side, a transplant was done within a month. It was Pam's sister who donated the kidney. From this point on, Pam's condition took a tremendous turn for the better. Her high blood pressure was more easily controlled iwth just one medication; there was reversal of Pam's retinopathy and Pam was now motivated! She educated herself and with her acquired knowledge of how to keep her blood sugars controlled, Pam opted to use the help of an insulin pump.

It has been five years since Pam's transplant. Pam married

Christopher, returned to school, received an R.N. degree in nursing and just on month ago delivered her second helathy son! Both of her pregnancies wer with no medical problems or complications from diabetes.

Her blood pressure and blood sugars were well controlled and there were no problems with retinopathy (her eyes).

The message from this story is manifold:

◆ Medical problems are preventable with good blood sugar control. This is evident in that Pam had no redevelopement of the complications in the five years since her transplant. It would have been better and less stressful if she had the wherewith all to prevent these problems in the first.

◆ Even if there are complications, it is not necessarily an indication of fate or doom. Pam had major problems, that were reversed with proper treatment, education, and motivation.

◆ Pam had Christopher and togehter they are a courageous couple. Pam is one of the few women in the world to have had two children after a kidney transplant.

◆ With good medical care, blood sugar control, women can lead healthy lives and know safe pregnancies, free of complications. It is my experience women with diabetes can do as well as women without diabetes.

Breastfeeding

Most of the women I've followed after childbirth chose to breastfeed their babies. From the diabetes control stand point, there is no reason not to breastfeed, as long as the mother is healthy and running good blood sugars.

24

Men and Diabetes:
The Problem of Sexual Dysfunction

Impotence

Impotence refers to the inability of a man to obtain an adequate erection of the penis during sexual intimacy. An occasional episode is not uncommon, but if it recurs frequently or becomes persistent, it needs further investigation. There are many possible medical as well as psychological causes of impotence. These causes should be closely investigated by a physician before diabetes is considered the culprit. Medication side effects, vascular diseases, multiple sclerosis, spinal cord disease, and thyroid disease should all be considered.

It should be known that impotence can be an initial manifestation of diabetes, as discussed in Chapter 4: "Subtle Signs of Diabetes." In a study (reported in the *Journal of the American Medical Association*, 244:2430), a group of 63 men with normal sexual function was compared with a group of 58 impotent men. It was found that 12% of the impotent men had glucose intolerance, whereas there were no cases of glucose intolerance in the group of men with normal sexual function. This tends to suggest that before psychological problems are considered a cause for impotence, a man should first make sure he doesn't have diabetes. As discussed below, treatment of diabetes may cure impotence.

It has been estimated in various studies that impotence occurs in between 10% and 50% of men with diabetes. Although psychological causes may certainly contribute to impotence in the man with diabetes, underlying complications related to the diabetes can often be the more clinically significant factors. There is no doubt in my mind (I'm not sure all authorities would agree) that the fatigue, loss of energy, and possible weight loss associated with prolonged periods of uncontrolled diabetes can most definitely sap a man of his libido or desire for sex and lead to transient episodes of impotence. In addition, poor control of diabetes may lead to infections of the penis and prostate gland, which could also contribute to impotence. I have seen many cases where improved diabetes control has cured these forms of impotence.

Before discussing the more chronic forms of impotence, it is important to understand that certain cases of impotence among men with diabetes may not be related to the diabetes itself, but may be a side-effects of medications or alcohol.

Cigarette smoking has been associated with erectile difficulties. Smokers have been found to have a higher incidence of sexual difficulties than non-smokers. Cigarette smoking may affect both the blood flow to the penis through the arteries necessary for erection and the blood flow from the veins. As a result, it may not only cause difficulties getting an erection, but the erection may not last as long. Secondly, drugs that are used to "get high" can affect sexual desire and performance. This is especially the case with marijuana and alcohol. Both can decrease libido and testosterone levels. Besides erectile difficulties, they may cause undesirable breast enlargement and decrease sperm production.

Finally, certain drugs that have valid therapeutic places in treating various medical problems may cause impotence as a side effect. These include many blood pressure medicines (antihypertensives), antidepressants, muscle relaxants, cholesterol lowering drugs, drugs used to reduce nausea, and anti-ulcer drugs (Tagamet® and Zantac®). All of these medicines exert their desired effects by altering either hormonal or nervous system response. If a man has become impotent as a result of taking one of these medications, it may be possible to reverse this effect. The impotence may he reversed by varying the dose, or trying a different (but therapeutically equivalent) drug.

The degree and length of an erection are also under hormonal and nervous system control. Unfortunately, one side effect of the alteration of these responses can be impotence. And as the man with diabetes gets older, there can be other reasons for impotence. Since an erection occurs by engorgement of the penis with blood, impaired blood flow caused by disease of the blood vessels (arteriosclerosis) is a fairly common cause of impotence. Even more common is diabetes neuropathy, a nerve disease that affects the arteries and veins that control blood flow to the penis. Arteriosclerosis and diabetes neuropathy generally occur in people with diabetes who have had poor control of their blood glucose levels over a period of several years.

A thorough evaluation by a physician can determine whether the cause of impotence is impairment of blood flow or the nervous system. This evaluation may include a penile nocturnal tumescence study (the disease-free man has an average of four erections associated with sexual dreams. The Tumescence Study measures the enlargement and hardness of the penis during these dreams per night lasting 15 to 60 minutes in the dream portion of his sleep). If tumescence does not occur, this may mean that medical reasons are causing it. Then a penile doppler which tests for adequacy of blood flow and nerve test such as a "Neurodiagnostic study" to study adequacy of nerve function can be done.

If it is proven that there is an organic or medical cause for impotence, this may in fact be a cause for relief for several reasons. For instance, when impotence first develops, marital discord may occur. A wife may feel rejected, or suspect her spouse of having a new woman. A man may feel threatened that his wife will leave him for a man who can better satisfy her. But when both partners are aware that the cause for the impotence is real and not because of loss of interest in either partner, there is a lessening of this emotional tension.

In addition, it's important to remember that sexual pleasure, intimacy and orgasm for both partners can take place even without intercourse. Ask Ann Landers about that in her survey of sexual satisfaction among women. Don't be afraid to reach out for help and explore new avenues. My beautiful fiancee, Becky bought us the book entitled "Mars and Venus, In the Bedroom" by John Gray and it has been a wonderful insightful growing tool for our relationship. However, if both partners prefer penile-vaginal intercourse, there are measures that will allow this. In a small percentage of these patients, there are medicines that will improve blood flow enough to allow for an erection. One of these medicines is called Yohimbine, which can be taken orally 3 times per day. If this fails, injections of medicines such as Papaverine, Regitine and/or Alprostadil directly into the corpora cavernosa of the penis cause the penile artery to dilate and an erection to occur.

With proper evaluation and education this therapy can be safe and effective but it is important for patients to be monitored closely. If impotence is caused by organic or medical reasons, which cannot be reversed, there are some external devices that will allow for the resumption of more satisfying sexual intercourse. These external devices are available in two types: entrapment or non entrapment devices.

The entrapment device, is an external vacuum device that is placed over the penis and an erection is achieved. After the penis is hard and firm, a band is placed over the base of the penis to entrap blood and maintain the erection. The external device is then removed from the erect penis. Since this is not a condom, this allows the man to have more sensation, which may allow sexual satisfaction to be a little more pleasurable for the man. One of my patients had been impotent for 3 years. After using it, he said that being able to resume sexual intimacy through intercourse with his wife made a difference of "night and day" in their relationship. The device is so simple and reliable that I would definitely recommend it for anyone interested in regaining potency prior to considering more invasive surgery.

There are a number of companies that make the entrapment device including: Vetco, Inc.,2928 6th Ave., South, Suite A, Birmingham, AL 35233 (1-800-827-8382); Performance Medical, P.O. Box 620, Berlin, N.J. 08009 (1-800-877-7420); ErecAid made by Osbon Medical Systems, P.O. Drawer 1478, Augusta, GA 30903 (1-800-438-8592); Response System, manufactured by Smith-Collins Pharmaceutical, 889 South Matlack Street, West Chester, PA (1 800-444-5748); and Post-T-Vac, Inc., P.O. Box 1436DF, Dodge City, KS 67801 (1-800-627-7434).

Finally, if the above methods are unsatisfactory, the man might benefit from penile prosthesis. There are several types that are now available, which are inserted by urologists. One young man I've treated says that sex became far better following penile implant than it was before he originally had the problem. His wife echoed his satisfaction. Lastly, if all medical reasons have been ruled out, counseling is an option I highly recommend.

There's Hope!

For any man who may have a problem with impotence and who wonders whether things will ever improve, all is not lost. Take encouragement from a man I've been treating who told me how he lost his sex drive for two to three years. He knew something was wrong because he found that as he lay in bed with his wife each night, he did not have to resort to reading religious literature, as he customarily had in the past, in order to avoid stimulation of his sexual desire. His wife did not seem to mind very much, thinking that five children was enough, but he began to wonder, and so he sought my opinion.

His medical history showed that he had developed diabetes over the years. However, he had not followed any special diet, and he had not paid much attention to how well his diabetes was being controlled. After listening to his story and evaluating his condition, I suggested that better control of his diabetes through proper diet and exercise might well bring back his potency. I am very happy to report that once he followed these recommendations, my patient had cause to resume his old habit of reading religious literature (even more so after the birth of their sixth child) as he lay with his wife each night.

Topical Cream for Erectile Dysfunction

A non-invasive therapeutic approach to helping diabetes patients suffering from erectile dysfunction is now in clinical development by International Medical Innovations, Inc. (Birmingham, AL). In this treatment, a small amount of the IMX-100 topical cream is applied directly to the penis, resulting in an erection in about ten minutes, and lasting from 30 to 45 minutes. While the firmness of the erection depends to some extent on the disease status of the patient, many have found it sufficient for resuming normal sexual activities.

Urologists working with IMX-100 consider it to have great potential as a first line of treatment for erectile dysfunction. The active ingredient in this medication has a long history of safe use as a cardiovascular medicine.

As this book goes to press, IMX-100 is undergoing the last stages of clinical trials. If all continues to go well, it should reach the U.S. marketplace by the end of 1997.

25

Diabetes After 50

Although more than 10% of people in their sixties develop diabetes, this form of the disease fortunately tends to be mild and uncomplicated. Concentrated carbohydrates may need to he restricted in the diet, but there should be little change in lifestyle for the older person with diabetes. Increasing physical exercise or activity to increase longevity may also help. Recent information indicates that as one ages, there tends to be some glucose intolerance so that blood sugars may run somewhat higher.

In other words, blood sugar levels that may be considered indicative of diabetes in a 20-year-old may be considered part of the normal aging process at age 70, as long as they are not excessive. To be more specific, most physicians would consider a 20-year-old patient a diabetic if he persistently had fasting blood sugars in the range of 130mg% to 140mg% or above, but would avoid this diagnosis if the patient were nearing 70. Although I would not necessarily label a 70-year-old with those blood sugars as a person with diabetes, I would probably offer him some advice. I would advise him against poor dietary habits and urge him to get what exercise he could. In addition, it would be important to have frequent medical checkups with particular attention to blood circulation, nervous system, and feet.

The onset of diabetes in the older person may coincide with a heart attack, gallbladder attack, or a number of other illnesses or infections. blood sugars may climb to 500mg% or more, and insulin may be needed to get them back to normal. Once the illness is over, and an appropriate diet, high in fiber, is begun, blood sugars may improve and insulin can frequently be discontinued. These patients should then be treated in the same way as people with glucose intolerance.

Another common problem concerns the patient who has developed high blood sugars in the 200 to 350mg% range, but who is otherwise well and has no major health problems. It is hard to convince such a patient that he needs insulin. Of course, diet and exercise should be tried first, and an attempt to control blood sugars with the help of the oral agents may also be worthwhile. If the blood sugars respond within several weeks, the pills can then be stopped. If, however, none of these methods are effective in controlling the blood sugar levels, insulin therapy should be considered, depending on age and other relevant factors. The goal of insulin therapy in this case is to control fasting blood sugars relatively well, allowing some elevation of blood sugar after meals. This approach is less harmful than one which attempts perfect control and risks hypoglycemia.

Without question, insulin is helpful to many patients in their sixties, seventies, or eighties. There are many patients who have had such poor diabetes control despite proper diet, exercise, and maximum dosage of oral agents that they look like they are literally dying of cancer or starvation (and feel as if they are, too). Insulin treatment for these patients frequently results in weight gain and increased strength and vigor.

For those patients who have had diabetes for several years, complications may be present. Since cases of diabetes vary so widely, it is impossible to discuss them individually within the scope of this book. Those people with long duration diabetes should already be well informed about their particular type of disease and need no further explanation here.

An 84 Year Old Woman with Diabetes, Takes the Plunge and Agrees to Insulin

One of the most fascinating ladies I have ever had the pleasure of meeting was 79-years-old when I met her. Her life had been full of adventure. She was acquainted with the Rockefellers and the Thompsons, she traveled a good deal, enjoyed occasional cocktails and even bet at the horse races. She had a loving circle of family and friends and enjoyed an active social life. During World War II she volunteered as a WAC and spent time in Alaska. There, she had the opportunity to drive the well-known Russian Communist, Vyacheslav Molotov (the U.S.S.R's foreign minister during the mid-fifties), around in a jeep. After the war she married a prestigious surgeon, continued to live in high society, and had three splendid children.

Her good life was marred only by frequent medical problems. By the time she saw me, she had been hospitalized 44 times for various ailments, none of which were related to diabetes. These included abdominal surgeries, a thyroid condition and a badly fractured arm. But the impact of all these medical problems on the rest of her life was hardly evident.

However, at the age of 79 she was beset with diabetes and was understandably shocked. She had heard all the terrible things that are frequently rumored to occur with diabetes. The end of life's road was not far away, and that was when our paths crossed.

Her family doctor had suggested that she see me, recommending me as a "that renowned, prominent diabetes specialist of South Jersey." After reviewing her history and giving her a physical examination, I impressed upon her that she was very well preserved despite her diabetes. I recommended that she not indulge her sweet tooth, cut down on the cocktails, take an oral hypoglycemic agent, and continue with her life as usual.

She did well over the next five years, but then, despite blood sugar readings only in the 130-to-260mg% range, she began losing ground. She got weak, tired, and began to lose weight. First she gave up the cocktails, but the final straw came when she had to give up the racetrack.

Circumstances suggested the possibility of underlying disease, even cancer. However, rather than put her through a series of elaborate and expensive tests, I suggested insulin, hoping it was only uncontrolled diabetes that needed correction. At age 84, she was not exactly titillated by the idea of going on insulin injections, but her common sense prevailed, and she agreed. With insulin injections she regained her strength and her zest for living and even returned to the racetrack. She recently died at age 95 years!

I'm not sure what her final winnings at the racetrack were! But this lady's story emphasizes that insulin can be a great help, no matter what a person's age. If you need insulin, don't fight it, even if you're over 50. See Maria's story next.

The Life of Maria –
An 87 Year Old Woman with Diabetes

In 1971 after a routine physical my Internist told me I had diabetes. I couldn't believe it - or rather I didn't want to believe it. It was summer and I had been drinking more sodas than usual and I felt that was the cause of there being sugar in my blood and urine, and the frequent urination was due to consuming too many liquids. However, on a return visit to the doctor and more tests 3 weeks later, I *had* to believe it. I thought it was the end for me because I was 60 years old and was about to retire. I had heard that diabetes was hereditary but there was no diabetes in my family. I still thought it was an error. My doctor told me I would have to make changes in my life style if I wanted to live. No cigarettes. That was easy - I wasn't a smoker. No more cocktails. I did have an occasional drink before dinner but I could do without it, no problem. But no sweets - that was different. My family had been in the candy business for almost a hundred years. I was accustomed to the best candy. It would be difficult, but I would do it. I loved life and I wanted to keep on living. So I did what I had to do. I got literature about diabetes, I learned about exchanges and the diabetes diet. It was fortunate that I like all vegetables and fruit and all good food. All I had to do was keep to the required amounts of food consumed. Cooking has always been a hobby of mine. I planted an herb garden and used different herbs to enhance the variety of things I cooked.

My physician passed away and there was no one in this

area who specialized in diabetes. Again, I was fortunate to learn there was a very good doctor who specialized in diabetes about an hour away. I made an appointment with Dr. Peter Lodewick. He was superb. Any problems that might appear - he was there to take care of them. Being a person with diabetes himself, he knew our problems. When machines became available to monitor blood sugar, I purchased one. I followed his advice and I felt well, and even though I was getting old, I lived and active life. When Dr. Lodewick left the area to work with people with diabetes in Birmingham, Alabama, I was devastated, but he had taught me well, so I need not have worried - but I missed him.

I have lived with diabetes for 26 years. If I live to my next birthday I will be 88 years old. I maintain a fairly large home, I cook good meals "from scratch", no prepared things. I take care of my herb garden, plus tomatoes and flowers. I do work at the hospital when I'm needed and serve on the Coalition for Diabetes Education in the county. I knit beautiful sweaters and enjoy having friends for meals. Many have said, "This can't be a diabetes meal. It's delicious". I also drive my car wherever I want to go. I lead an active life for anyone my age. I have outlived my children and 3 husbands, none of whom had diabetes.

If you are diagnosed with diabetes, don't worry. It is not a death sentence. Learn to follow the diabetes exchange list and eat right. Get a monitor and learn to adjust your insulin accordingly. Have a good doctor and follow his advice and you can live to be in your 80's or even 90's. Who knows - I may even live to celebrate 100!

Maria Aimone, 1996

26

Complications

This is the one chapter of the book that I wish I did not have to write. Complications unfortunately can occur with diabetes. When insulin was discovered in 1921, doctors hoped that the "cure" for diabetes had been found. Certainly, insulin does prevent the rapid progression of the disease in insulin-dependent diabetes. However, we have found that even with the benefits of insulin, complications can still occur. The death of the great Brooklyn Dodgers baseball player, Jackie Robinson, the first black athlete to break into major league baseball, was attributed to diabetes complications. Cases such as this remind us that all diabetes may be susceptible to complications, and that insulin as we know it today is not a "cure" for diabetes. The *Diabetes Control and Complications Trial* (DCCT) as discussed in the research chapter definitely proved that good blood sugar control as well as blood pressure control can slow down or prevent most of the diabetes complications.

What are the complications and how do they develop? In general, the blood vessels take the brunt of the problems associated with diabetes. The blood vessels in the eyes, kidneys, nervous system, heart and legs can all experience complications from diabetes. There are two different types of blood vessel disease: small vessel disease and large vessel disease. Small vessel disease involves the eyes, kidneys, and nervous system, whereas large vessel disease involves the legs and heart.

Eye Complications

Small vessel disease is most striking in the eye. In the retina of the eye there are many veins and arteries that are

visible by looking through the pupil with a physician's oph-
thalmoscope. When diabetes affects these vessels, the veins
become enlarged and twisted, and the arteries become narrowed. Microaneurysms occur, which are dilatations in the
smallest vessels that lie between the arteries and veins.
Associated with aneurysms are small, dot-sized hemorrhages.
Occasionally, white or yellow spots are also seen. These dots,
called *exudates*, may consist of dead eye tissue that results
from the impairment of the blood vessels that supply the eye
with the necessary nutrients. The eye changes discussed so
far are referred to as benign retinopathy because, for the most
part, they do not lead to loss of vision.

However, as diabetes progresses (particularly when the
diabetes has been poorly controlled) there can be leakage of
fluid from the blood vessels and an accumulation of the fluid
in the retina (*retinal edema*), which can result in loss of vision.
In my practice, I have seen this condition many times. In
some cases, when I feared that a patient's vision would
continue to get worse, I found drastic improvement after the
patient started to take better care of himself by controlling
blood sugars and abstaining from alcohol. Good control of
diabetes is essential to curbing the development of these
complications.

Another severe retinal disease is *proliferative retinopathy*,
where the blood vessels of the retina proliferate (the reason is
unknown) forming new blood vessels. These new blood vessels tend to bleed into and behind the area called the *vitreous
humor* of the eye (it is the clear tissue located behind the lens),
causing impaired vision, retinal detachment, and even blindness. Up to eight percent of people with diabetes may develop this type of severe retinopathy. Here, too, many medical
professionals find that the more severe types of eye disease
are rarely seen in patients keeping their diabetes under good
control.

If proliferative retinopathy does develop, it is possible
that partial loss of vision and blindness can be prevented
with laser treatment. A major study, called the Diabetic
Collaborative Study, was conducted in the 1970s by the

National Eye institute. In this study, patients with proliferative retinopathy had one of their eyes treated with a laser
beam to prevent bleeding of the abnormal vessels, while the
other eye was not treated. Results of the study indicated that
the eye treated with laser therapy had far less vision loss than
the eye that did not receive laser treatment.

Because of the eye complications associated with diabetes,
you should have your eyes checked by a doctor who is experienced in treating retinopathy caused by diabetes at least
once a year. It is important for the people with diabetes to
realize that serious changes in the eye can occur without any
significant visual disturbances before the sudden onset of
blindness. If the eyes are checked regularly, the problems can
be identified before vision is impaired, laser treatment can be
given, and blindness can be prevented.

The following table lists people who are at an increased
risk of developing retinopathy and should be checked with
greater frequency, preferably by an ophthalmologist or retinal
specialist.

Persons	Frequency of Eye Check
With 15 years of diabetes	At Least Yearly
Children	By age 13, then yearly or more, depending on presence of retinopathy.
Pregnant	Prepregnancy and at least every trimester. Every 4-6 weeks if retinopathy is present.
Hypertensive	At diagnosis and at least yearly even if retinopathy is not initially present.
With retinopathy present	Every 4-6 months.
With sudden vision loss	Immediately, unless treating doctor can explain it by fluctuating blood sugar control.
On medicine for other serious medical disorders.	Soon afterward.

A final word about *cataracts*. Cataracts are changes in the lens that may eventually obscure vision. All people as they get older get cataracts. Only some of them will have their vision affected significantly by cataracts. Persons with diabetes are included in this category. They get cataracts too, generally at an earlier age. Many physicians feel that poor diabetes control tends to accelerate cataract development, and research supports their thinking. Therefore, two important points to follow:

◆ Keep diabetes as well under control as possible; this will help slow down the development of cataracts

◆ If and when cataracts develop, remember that there is advanced surgery, now available, that can remedy the situation; this includes intraocular lens implantation, a procedure that effectively restores vision. Diabetes should not be a barrier to this surgery.

Kidney Complications

Just as diabetes affects the eyes, it can also affect the kidneys. If there are eye changes attributed to diabetes, there is a moderate chance that kidney changes are also present. The kidneys contain a vast network of blood vessels, and in people with diabetes, these blood vessels may become damaged and may leak protein. This condition is signalled by protein in the urine, called *proteinuria*, or microalbumin. Diabetes can be present for less than 10 years when proteinuria occurs. Once it does occur, it is not uncommon to find blood vessels in the kidney becoming sclerotic (hardened and narrowed). As these changes occur, hypertension may also result. Eventually, the kidneys may fail. Because of the serious implications of kidney disease, it is extremely important for the people with diabetes to have close medical attention. Some recent studies have demonstrated that kidney disease can be prevented from progressing if it is detected early enough. One way of diagnosing early kidney disease is with a test for "microalbumin" in the urine. Patients with diabetes should probably have this test every 6 to 12 months. The use of some medications and good diabetes control have been shown to reverse this microalbumin.

Hypertension and kidney infections are particularly important warning signs of a diseased kidney. Treatment of these disorders may slow down the progression of kidney disease. Current research also seems to indicate that good control of blood sugar and a low protein diet helps retard kidney degeneration. Some of the medicines used to control blood pressure, the "Ace Inhibitors" may also effectively retard kidney disease. The "Ace Inhibitors" are generally used in people for high blood pressure but may also be useful even in people with normal blood pressure. Discuss this with your doctor. Blood pressure levels as over as 135/85 mmHg are now considered high.

Nervous System Complications

Diabetes neuropathy is the general term used to describe a disease of the nerves. Nerve cells are very long cells emanating from the spinal cord or brain. Since the nerves connect to all the tissues of the body, diabetes neuropathy can affect the feet, joints, heart, muscles, stomach, intestines and bladder.

When the feet are affected, loss of sensation usually occurs. This can start very subtly with numbness or "cold feet." As the neuropathy progresses, complete loss of pain sensation sometimes occurs. When this happens, a person may be unaware that a cut, a blister or even an infection is present until it has progressed to such a degree that it requires hospital care. This condition can be the precursor of gangrene, as discussed later in this chapter. Any patient with neuropathy of the feet should take all possible precautions, as outlined in Chapter 22, "Foot Care."

When neuropathy involves the muscular system, it can result in weakness, clumsiness, muscle wasting and even paralysis. Sometimes the paralysis involves only one muscle, such as an eye muscle (possibly resulting in double vision).

Frequently, however, this type of neuropathy is associated with inflammation of the nerves and therefore is called neuritis. The pain in this condition can be excruciating. The most severe cases of *neuritis* that I have seen occurred in patients whose diabetes had been out of control for a long period of time, and many have had a long history of excessive alcohol consumption. It is possible that a vitamin deficiency may also contribute to the neuropathy.

Paradoxically, it is not uncommon to see neuropathy temporarily exacerbated when attempts to control the diabetes are made. This sometimes occurs just after insulin therapy is started, so that the patient may even blame insulin for the condition. For the physician involved, this situation is particularly difficult because the patient can get discouraged if he doesn't see immediate improvement; yet if attempts to control the diabetes are not made and sustained, the health of the patient is in serious jeopardy. In general, the condition stabilizes after four to six months of good control, and the neuritis pain becomes more tolerable. In the meantime, some medications (amitriptylene, phenytoin, Fenfluphenazine, Prozac, tegretol, and Neurontin) can be used with varying degrees of success. Vitamins such as high doses of Vitamin C (1500mg/d) and folic acid may also help. Synthetic nerve growth factor shows promises as a way of relieving this condition.

Neuropathy can also affect the autonomic nervous system, which controls blood pressure responses, heart rate, heart contraction, bladder emptying, stomach and intestinal function and sexual performance. When blood pressure responses are affected by diabetes neuropathy, an abrupt fall in blood pressure may occur with standing. This results in decreased circulation of blood to the brain. Dizziness and even loss of consciousness can occur. When neuropathy affects the heart rate, there may not be an appropriate increase in the rate of the heart beat upon exercise, and again a blackout can occur. Impairment of heart rate and heart contractions could cause heart failure (which means the heart does not pump blood properly), especially after a heart attack.

Neuropathy affecting the urinary bladder causes delays in

emptying. Normally, it takes 200-to-300 milliliters (6-to-10 ounces) of urine in the bladder before a person feels the urge to void. With neuropathy of the bladder, however, this urge to void is lost, and the bladder may fill up with as much as one quart of urine and then not empty fully. This condition can lead to bladder infections.

Finally, when neuropathy affects the stomach and intestines, it can cause a variety of symptoms. Poor stomach emptying may result in distention of the stomach and periods of vomiting. A drug, metoclopramide (Reglan) or cisapride (Propulsid), has been partially successful in treating this problem. Constipation and diarrhea can also occur with neuropathy of the gastrointestinal tract and may require medical attention.

Complications of the Large Blood Vessels

Most of the above complications involving the eye, kidney, and nerves are triggered by small blood vessel disease. When diabetes affects the larger blood vessels, it may affect the legs, heart and aorta. When the larger blood vessels in the legs are affected, arteriosclerosis, or hardening of the arteries can occur because of the decreased blood flow. Arteriosclerosis may initially manifest itself by changes in skin texture, loss of leg hair and discoloration of the skin on the legs with blue mottling. As the arteriosclerosis progresses, cramping of the leg muscles occurs with walking or exercise. This condition is referred to as *intermittent claudication* and may limit exercise. A medication called Trental may help in this situation.

Finally, *gangrene*, the most feared complication of diabetes, may occur. Gangrene is literally the wasting away of tissue due to a lack of an adequate blood supply. Neuropathy and infection usually accompany gangrene, and may ultimately lead to loss of a limb. My experience with gangrene is that in a large number of cases, neglect of wounds is at least partially responsible. This is because, if neuropathy does develop (and it may not in all people), many times patients are unaware that they have these wounds and therefore unknowingly neglect them. That's why it's so important to inspect the feet carefully each day and to treat fungal infections early. When a person with diabetes has a foot wound, extreme care under a doctor's supervision should ensue. Hospitalization should strongly be considered if redness and foot swelling are present. I believe that most cases of amputation could have been prevented by proper initial care of a simple wound.

Although the most feared complication is gangrene, the most life-threatening complication is heart disease. People with diabetes have a much higher incidence of heart disease than the general population. In fact, if it weren't for heart disease, it is believed that non-insulin-dependent people with diabetes would live as long as people without diabetes. If a woman develops heart disease before menopause, there is a higher than average chance that she will have diabetes, whether or not it has manifested itself before hand.

Why people with diabetes have a greater incidence of heart disease is not fully established, but several areas of research seem to indicate that good control of diabetes can make a substantial difference. It has recently been found that if glycohemoglobin results are high, indicating that the control of diabetes is poor, there will often be an elevation of fats, cholesterol, and triglycerides in the blood. In addition, the HDL (high density lipoprotein or "good cholesterol") level in the blood, which serves as a protective factor against heart disease, is lower when diabetes control is poor.

Hypertension is another factor that may be responsible for the increased chance of heart disease in the person with diabetes. Individuals with diabetes have a higher incidence of hypertension, possibly because of kidney involvement, or because they have an associated condition of *essential hypertension*, which is common among the general population. In either case, the hypertension should be treated. Just as diabetes can aggravate arteriosclerosis and kidney disease, so can untreated hypertension. There are now some new medications that have become available that are effective in controlling blood pressure without as many side-effects, in particular, "Ace Inhibitors" and "calcium channel blockers."

Cigarette Smoking

As long as I am discussing factors that influence the course of heart disease, I should address the issue of cigarette smoking. First of all, in people with both diabetes without diabetes, cigarettes have an adverse effect of arteries, contributing to arteriosclerosis. There are three main arteries to the heart called the *coronary arteries*, and arteriosclerosis affects these arteries, causing *coronary artery disease*. Cigarette smoking also affects other major arteries, such as those arteries in the brain and legs. There has been evidence that cigarette smoking has adverse effects on the small blood vessels, too. For instance, studies seem to indicate that people with diabetes who smoke have a higher incidence of retinopathy than nonsmokers with diabetes. Cigarette smoking is hazardous to one's health, and especially to the health of the individual with diabetes.

Heart Disease

The typical symptom of heart disease is *angina pectoris*, which means pain in the chest. However, pain tends to vary in degree, location and type. It may be a sharp pain, a tightness, a shortness of breath or a sensation of gas in the chest similar to indigestion. Sometimes, it can be located in other areas besides the chest, such as in the jaw, arm or elbow. It is frequently triggered by exercise or intense emotion. Another indication of possible heart disease is heart failure. Symptoms of heart failure include fatigue, cough and shortness of breath. I have seen heart failure go undiagnosed many times, with a cough being dismissed as symptomatic of a cold or bronchitis. The cough and shortness of breath, particularly occur at night, making it difficult to lie flat.

Finally, there are some people with diabetes who don't develop most of the symptoms associated with heart disease, particularly the symptoms of angina pectoris (chest pain) despite the fact that they do indeed have heart disease. These patients have what is called *silent heart disease*, and for some reason do not experience angina. One possible explanation is the fact that neuropathy could have impaired the nerves in the heart that transmit pain. It is very critical to be on the alert for this asymptomatic heart disease, particularly if exercise is recommended as a form of treatment, since people with diabetes must exercise with caution if heart disease is present. To diagnose this silent heart disease, a stress or exercise electrocardiogram should be performed. I recommend this test for any person with diabetes over the age of 40, especially if diabetes has been present for several years.

Find Out More!

Because this chapter only touches on the complications of diabetes, it would be worthwhile for the reader to learn much more about these complications by writing the American Diabetes Association for literature, or by obtaining material from a local library or bookstore (I've listed some sources of information in Chapter 32, "Recommended Readings.") Although I have heard many people with diabetes say they are not interested in hearing about the complications of diabetes, their failure to learn about them could prove dangerous, as in the case of Jackie Robinson. By knowing more about possible complications, it is concluded that exercise, proper diet and good diabetes control are the best ways to prevent the development of serious complications. In the meantime we will search for even better treatments for diabetes. For more of the latest information read the Research chapter, also.

27

What To Do When Ill

Knowing how to take care of yourself when you are ill is, understandably, a vital part of keeping your diabetes under control. With the proper knowledge, you should have little fear of developing either diabetes coma with acidosis or coma from hypoglycemia.

Illness, even a minor one, often triggers elevation of blood sugar levels. For this reason, insulin-dependent people with diabetes often need more insulin, and those people with diabetes who normally control their disease without insulin may need doses of regular insulin during the course of their illness. Thus, many people with diabetes who don't normally take insulin might become familiar with the material in this chapter in case sickness necessitates insulin use.

Contrary to popular belief, "plenty of juices and fluids" is not good advice for a person with diabetes who is ill unless he knows exactly how these fluids are going to affect blood sugar levels. Consult your physician in this regard. Sugar and acetone tests should help you monitor the effects of your illness. If you are very sick, it is a good idea to have a friend or relative stay with you.

Sick Day Rules for Type I Insulin-Dependent Diabetes

If you have Type I insulin-dependent diabetes, the most important rule during illness is never omit your daily insulin dose. Test your blood or urine for sugar at least four times per day (before meals and at bedtime) and record the results. Depending on the seriousness of the illness and other results of the tests, more frequent testing may be required. You should also test your urine for acetone, especially if you are very ill. If you have negative urine sugar results or your blood sugar is under 180mg% but high acetone results, you many need to eat more carbohydrates. <u>Call your physician, letting him know the results of your blood and/or urine tests</u>, the amount of your usual insulin dose, and the extent of your fever or illness.

If you are experiencing nausea, vomiting, and are passing a lot of urine, take clear soups or salty broths every hour or so. These will help replace valuable salts and minerals. Also, make note of whether your tongue feels moist or dry. A dry tongue is a very important sign, indicating that your body is losing more fluids than you are replacing.

If you are able to eat your normal diet and blood sugar is over 200mg% or your urine tests are consistently positive for sugar, you may need supplementary regular insulin. You will also definitely <u>need extra Regular insulin</u> if you are eating less than usual, experiencing nausea and vomiting, find your blood sugar high, or find sugar and acetone in your urine. The dose of regular insulin will vary according to many factors, especially the degree of the illness, the stage or type of diabetes and the amount of acetone. Follow the judgment of your physician. In general, the following rules apply:

◆ Take your usual dose of insulin
◆ You may take additional regular insulin according to the schedule on the following page if there are high levels of blood sugar and, sugar and acetone in the urine:

If you are very sick and have a high urine acetone reading, more frequent blood and urine testing and more insulin may be necessary. See the discussion about ketoacidosis in Chapter 10: "Low and High Blood Sugar Reactions: Hypoglycemia and Ketoacidosis," and discuss these recommendations with your doctor.

If you can't eat the foods in your regular diet, attempt to follow the diet outlined below (you can substitute any of the foods below, if necessary, with equivalent foods). This diet

Doses of Additional Regular Insulin				
Blood Sugar (mg%)	7 AM	11:30 AM	5 PM	9 PM
If you take fewer than 16 units a day, total (to include more than one kind of insulin)				
Over 240	4 U reg	4 U reg	4 U reg	4 U reg
120-240	2 U reg	2 U reg	2 U reg	2 U reg
Less than 120	0	0	0	0
If you take 16-40 Units a day, total –				
Over 240	6 U reg	6 U reg	6 U reg	6 U reg
120-240	4 U reg	4 U reg	4 U reg	4 U reg
Less than 120	0	0	0	0
If you take more than 40 Units a day total –				
Over 240	10 U reg	10 U reg	10 U reg	10 U mg
120-240	6 U reg	6 U reg	6 U reg	6 U reg
Less than 120	0	0	0	0

contains approximately 1200 calories. Although it may contain fewer calories than your usual diet, you probably don't have to worry about low blood sugar since your illness elevates the blood sugar, as mentioned in the beginning of this chapter. That is also why it is important not to skip your insulin dose. When insulin is skipped the blood sugar can go high even without eating, because the liver makes insulin.

Sick Day Diet

<u>Breakfast</u>
    1/2 c applesauce
    1 poached egg on toast with butter *or* 1 oz. American cheese on toast
    Tea with lemon

10 AM
1/2 c cereal
1/2 c milk
Tea

Lunch
Broth (clear)
2 oz. cottage cheese with 1/2 c canned dietetic fruit
Saltines with butter
Tea with lemon

3 PM
3/4 c orange juice
Toast with butter

Dinner
2 oz. slice chicken or small omelet
Baked potato with butter
Tomato juice
Regular Jello

Bedtime
1/2 c apple juice or 1/2 c canned dietetic fruit
Toast or 5 Saltines
Tea with lemon

Cases of food poisoning or severe vomiting and diarrhea (gastroenteritis) are special instances when you may want to be cautious about taking your full dose of insulin. If the urine tests are negative for sugar and acetone, and the blood sugar is under 120mg%, you may take one-half to three-quarters of the usual dose and possibly take the rest when your appetite improves. If the tests are positive for sugar and acetone and the blood sugar is over 200mg%, the whole dose of insulin should probably be taken. If, in either of the above cases, vomiting or nausea continues for more than four hours, you may very well have more than just food poisoning or a virus, and you should contact your physician.

Sick Day Rules For Non-Insulin-Dependent Type 2 Diabetes

For people who generally do not require insulin for control, most mild illnesses will not cause blood sugars to go higher. However, occasionally marked blood sugar elevations will occur, especially with more serious illnesses. If the blood sugars do go significantly above 240mg% and you are experiencing symptoms of high blood sugar, a call to your physician is warranted, especially if the urine is checked for ketones and found to be high. So make sure to check the urine ketones. Occasionally, certain illnesses may require insulin use at least temporarily. Once the illness is over, insulin requirements may stop.

For people who are on some oral (pill) medicine for blood sugar control, the blood sugar should be checked if nausea is present. If it is under 120mg%, it may not be advisable to take all the oral diabetes medication so that low blood sugar does not result. Check this out with your doctor. Follow the same eating guideline for Type I diabetes.

28

Traveling with Diabetes

The urge to travel is intrinsic in all of us. We love it! We desire to move, to see, to go elsewhere, and learn about faraway cultures different from our own. It is mind-expanding. It sparks creativity, as we relax from our everyday world. Having diabetes does not change this adventurous spirit and should not prevent exploration of the world around us and giving us a chance to play.

Too often, however, people with diabetes give up their desire to travel and confine themselves to their homes, leaving only for necessities such as food and work. Their reasons for doing so may include ignorance of diet flexibility, fear of illness, or an assumption that travel always involves complex arrangements or they may not be well controlled or in good physical shape. The following points are some practical tips that should make traveling less threatening and more enjoyable.

Pack early. Make sure you bring along the blood testing paraphernalia to keep you abreast of how well your blood glucose control is. It is better to know for sure what your blood sugar is than to guess at it so you can avoid both low and high blood sugar reactions. I have been fooled myself more than once by finding my blood sugars surprisingly high when traveling despite the fact that I was eating less. Whether it is the sitting around in a car, plane, or train that make it high or just the excitement is somewhat difficult to say. In cases such as these, I frequently have to cut my carbohydrates to prevent high blood sugar. Make sure you take along your urine ketone tests. If these are high, this may be an indication to take extra Regular insulin, especially if illness should occur.

Know your diet well. Consult your doctor or dietician if you have any questions. They should be able to help you choose the right foods, particularly if you are traveling to foreign countries where the basic foods are entirely different from those to which you are accustomed. Go to restaurants serving foods suitable to your diet. Health food, vegetarian, and seafood restaurants should provide you with the essentials, but you must remember not to overdo a good thing. The typical American restaurant serves an overabundance of food, so when half-orders are not available, do not feel compelled to eat every thing on the plate.

Remember to avoid fried foods, excess butter and cream. Request a side order of dressing for your salad and a plain baked potato (without sour cream or butter) or other suitable bread substitutions. Although you don't want to eat excessively while on a trip, one or two meals per week in which you allow yourself to eat somewhat more heavily than normal should not cause much trouble. A little extra exercise on those days will help burn up the extra calories and keep the blood sugar down.

As for obtaining food while traveling by plane, most airlines are quite accommodating. If you are scheduling a long trip, an advance call to the airline will usually assure you of food that suits your diet. Even in cases when it is not possible to call in advance, most of the meals served aboard planes should not be much different from your usual diet. You should carry some food with you in case of unexpected delays, although in today's world it would be unusual not to have acceptable food readily available in such a situation.

For people with diabetes on insulin, a more than adequate insulin supply should be on hand in case part of it becomes lost. Insulin should be carried on your person, not in luggage, where it can be affected by temperature changes. It need not be refrigerated and can be easily kept in your pocket. A small change in insulin dosage may be necessary during a day of heavy traveling or if the time change through which you are traveling exceeds four hours. It is wise to discuss this with your doctor before your trip.

Jet lag is a common problem for all plane travellers to content with. It can cause irritability, fatigue, aching muscles and digestive disorders but so can poor diabetes control. So make sure diabetes control is good and take plenty of fresh, distilled water during the trip.

Maintaining your diet when traveling by van is very easy since a van has plenty of storage room for food. Automobile travel may mean stopping more frequently, but again, you should have food in the car in case of traffic delays. Highway travel is convenient because of the many food facilities along the roadside. The big problem here is resisting the temptation of constantly available food. Remember, letting blood sugar run high by overeating may exhaust your energies and make your trip much less enjoyable.

When traveling by ship, it is important that you avoid seasickness, which can greatly aggravate your diabetes and cause other medical problems. Dramamine (dimenhydrinate) or a similar medication may prevent this problem.

"Traveler's diarrhea" is another disorder that may occur, especially in those traveling long distances from home. This condition is thought to be caused by bacteria in some foods, or simply by a drastic change in diet. Bottled rather than tap water should be used whenever possible to avoid possible reactions to various water purification methods. It may be worth having your doctor prescribe an antibiotic if you are traveling to locales where diarrhea is known to be a problem. You might also want to bring along medicines to control nausea and vomiting, such as trimethobenzamide (or Tigan), or Bonine, as well as medicines that alleviate diarrhea, such as loperamide (Imodium) or diphenoxylate (Lomotil), and Pepto Bismol for abdominal cramping and nausea.

Remember to bring some form of identification on your trip that states you are a person with diabetes. If you are traveling to a foreign country, it is also wise to contact the American embassy in that country and get the names of English-speaking doctors. Write or call Intermedic for a list of English speaking doctors in your destination country, 777 Third Avenue, New York, NY, 10017, 1-212-486-8974.

In short, diabetes is no reason to inhibit travel. By knowing some basic information and taking some practical precautions, you can travel without substantial difficulties just like Romeo and Juliet.

29

Alcohol's Effects

Alcohol can relieve tensions, complement a gourmet meal and add to the conviviality of a social gathering. In excess, however, it can be deeply destructive. There is a wide range of attitudes about alcohol consumption. Some doctors strictly forbid the slightest alcohol consumption, while others are more flexible and adjust their attitudes to the needs and conditions of each particular person.

Ten percent of the U.S. population tend to consume too much alcohol. Excessive alcohol consumption can result in impairment of mental faculties, uncontrolled appetites, malnutrition, and personality changes. These consequences can eventually affect interpersonal relationships both at home and work, possibly leading to marital difficulties or the loss of a fine job.

The person with diabetes must be even more cautious with alcohol since large amounts of alcohol can complicate diabetes, making proper control very difficult. Although drinks (for example gin, vodka, bourbon, scotch and dry wine) are not carbohydrates, proteins, or fats, they do contain calories that must be accounted for in the diet. Despite the calories, alcohol does not contain the necessary minerals and vitamins needed by the body. It is very important not to "substitute" straight alcohol for a bread and fruit exchange (as some physicians previously recommended) because of its lack of nutrients and because such a substitution could greatly reduce blood sugar levels.

A full understanding of alcohol's effects is particularly critical for Type I insulin-dependent diabetes. A few drinks can reduce mental alertness, sometimes causing a delayed meal. A delayed meal combined with the fact that alcohol can inhibit gluconeogenesis (the liver's formation of glucose from noncarbohydrates) can lead to hypoglycemia and result in the loss of consciousness. With alcohol on the breath, this hypoglycemia may be mistaken for drunkenness, and this misconception could delay necessary treatment. People have been placed in jail with the presumption that they are drunk rather than hypoglycemic.

Drinking enough alcohol to cause nausea, vomiting, or a "hangover" may greatly interfere with proper diabetes control since dehydration and reduced food intake can induce ketoacidosis. Further more, continual excessive alcohol intake can damage the nerves, causing pain in the legs and feet (neuritis), reduced reflexes, muscle weakness, or even paralysis —symptoms which can mimic the onset of diabetes neuropathy. In turn, alcohol can worsen diabetes neuropathy when it does occur. Some of the most serious cases of diabetes neuropathy that I have seen occurred in people with a long history of uncontrolled diabetes compounded by prolonged, heavy alcohol intake.

Another troublesome effect of alcohol is frequently seen in patients using the oral antidiabetic agent Diabinese. In some patients, alcohol combined with Diabinese causes flushing, nausea, and "hot flash" sensations. The mechanism behind these symptoms is not well understood. However, paradoxically it is interesting to note that patients who suffer from these disturbing side effects do not usually suffer some of the chronic complications that are seen in diabetes.

Calories in Alcoholic Beverages

I have seen so many patients who are completely ignorant of the calories in alcoholic beverages that it no longer surprises me. Patients state that they maintain their 1200 calorie diet perfectly and wonder why their diabetes is not controlled, not taking into consideration the caloric content of the alcohol they drink. I know of one patient in particular who kept to his 1200 calorie diet except for one thing—he drank a case of beer every day. When he eliminated beer from his diet, he lost weight, he could stop using the oral hypoglycemic agent prescribed to him, and he was able to control his diabetes.

The caloric content of alcoholic beverages varies considerably. You may remember from the diet section of this book that carbohydrates have 4 calories per gram, proteins have 4 calories per gram, and fats have 9 calories per gram. Alcohol is metabolized differently from carbohydrates, proteins and fats, and has approximately 7 calories per gram. In addition, there are varying amounts of carbohydrates and sometimes small amounts of proteins in the different alcoholic beverages.

To simplify things, the American Diabetes Association has recently published an alcohol exchange list, reprinted on the following pages. This list does not include the sweet dessert wines or the liqueurs (most of which have more than 30% sugar and are high in alcohol content as well), which should be used cautiously, if at all. In general, most of the dry white wines include Chablis, Chenin Blanc, Pinot Noir, and Zinfandel. Dry red wines include the Burgundies, Beaujolais's, and red table wines. If there is any taste of sweetness, the wine should be consumed in less than 3-ounce quantities and should possibly be substituted for a fruit exchange, which brings me to the issue of mixed drinks.

Type of Alcohol	Ounces	Calories	Carbohydrate (g)	Exchanges
Rum, whiskey, gin, vodka				
42 proof	1 1/2	50	–	1 fat
80 proof	1 1/2	97	–	2 fats
100 proof	1 1/2	124	–	3 fats
Beer	12	170	16	1 bread, 2 fats
Diet beer or Light beer	12	96	–	2 fats
Wine				
Dry table wine	4	90		0-3 2 fats
Dry sherry	2	75	0-2	1 1/2 fats

It is not uncommon for people to mix a little juice with an alcoholic beverage in order to mask the bitter taste of alcohol. One such common drink is the Screwdriver, a blend of orange juice and vodka. The problem with this is twofold: first, people drink it as if it were plain orange juice; and second, the ease with which it is drunk may cause a double jeopardy: as the blood sugar is rapidly climbing, so is the blood alcohol content. However, if such beverages can be kept to a minimum, it may be reasonable to substitute an exchange or two in the diet depending on what is added to the alcohol in the beverage. A Screwdriver would be equivalent to one or more fruit exchanges, depending on the amount of orange juice. Beer might be substituted for one to two bread exchanges. Again, I caution you, just because your diet may allow 9 bread exchanges, you should not substitute 6 or 7 beers—the nutritional content is simply not the same!

I conclude, therefore, by saying that for those people who can enjoy an occasional drink, and not more than two light drinks on any day, it is likely that this minimal amount of alcohol will not have much effect on the diabetes. For those so inclined (providing they have the approval of their physicians), alcohol may be considered a cherished commodity, available to enliven the social and amicable spirits. To them: "Skoal!" To the nondrinkers: "Skoal!" as well.

Occasions When the Doctor Takes a Drink

Although I am acutely aware of the adverse effects of extreme alcohol consumption in the person with diabetes and person without diabetes alike, I do occasionally consume spirits. It is not unknown for me to celebrate a hard fought tennis victory with a beer to replenish the fluid deficiency from heavy exercise. I certainly will lift a glass of champagne to ring in the New Year or to offer a toast at a wedding celebration. Even a glass of dry, low-calorie wine can be seen passing my lips as I relax at home with my family in the evening.

30

Research – Quest for a Cure

Diabetes, Diabetes, O' Wherefore
Do you come...
Is it just food or fat that turns my health to bum
Diabetes, Diabetes, Wherefore
Do you come...
Is it just a virus in the air
that turns my health to fair

Exercise, proper diet, appropriate insulin dosage and general good health help to reduce the risk of diabetes complications, but the possibility still remains that complications will occur. Research is needed to expand our understanding of diabetes and to enable us to treat the disease more effectively. Current research is very active, and there is good reason to believe that some of the questions about this complicated disease will soon be answered.

Research on Good Diabetes Control

Does good diabetes control make a difference? Throughout this book, we have talked about the need to get as good blood sugar control as possible. Its value in pregnancy can't be denied, and we know that good control invariably makes the average person feel better than when the blood sugar is out of control. He or she is stronger, better-looking, more energetic. In addition, patients with good control on the average fare better with respect to all vascular complications than those who have poor control. To illustrate better what I am suggesting, I would like to say that if you take 100 people with good control, maybe 8 or 10 will get the bad vascular complications—compared to 100 people with poor control, where 18 or 20 will get complications. This can be looked at in two ways: People with good control do better statistically with regard to diabetes complications than those with poor control. But, on the other hand, an individual with good control may still get the complications, and there are many people with poor control who may not get complications at all. This being the case, some people with diabetes may say, "Why try?" My argument follows that statistically a person who gives up on control is taking a greater risk. In fact, it has been my impression that many patients I've seen with bad control who have begun to get complications, have reversed or at least slowed down those complications by changing their ways and gaining control of their blood sugar. The following describes such a case:

Renegade Becomes a Religious Missionary

I was referred a young fellow, 18-years-old, who had only had diabetes for five years (onset at age 13 years). He was a real renegade, causing considerable havoc at home by abusing his body and diabetes with a terrible combination of beer, alcohol and drugs. Where I first saw him at age 18, he was already experiencing significant changes in his retina, which is unusual in such a young person with only five years of diabetes. As he describes it, by the grace of God he became a born-again Christian, and a miracle resulted. His life was transformed. He decided it was about time he stopped causing such a ruckus for his family and himself. In addition to all the other changes that resulted, he chose to take better care of his diabetes.

Twelve years after the change in this young man's life allowed him to enter into the religious ministry and get married. He has found that the enjoyment he got from the recklessness of his teenage years cannot compare to the great joy he's derived from his transformed life. Not only has his personal life improved, but his retinopathy regressed, and the threat of imminent vision loss disappeared.

I have seen other patients with kidney, eye or neuropathic complications experience a regression or at least a slowed progression and a relatively stable condition that lasted for many years, because they cared for themselves with good diet and good control. However, many other doctors are not so sure that a reversal is likely once the signs of a complication exist. They say (and I agree), that it would be better to prevent the development of complications in the first place. Nevertheless, the general consensus among all of us is that good control is better than poor control.

The question is: Does very strict control—keeping the blood sugars as close to normal as possible (60-to-120mg%) — make a difference? For a person with diabetes, absolutely perfect control is practically impossible given that human beings are not perfect, and the methods we have of emulating the natural workings of the nondiabetic human body aren't so precise as to allow perfect control all the time. Extraordinary measures are needed if a person with diabetes is to have perfect control. However, the painstaking care needed to get perfect or strict control may not prevent the complications of diabetes any better than just fair to good control. So why, you may ask, put all the time and energy into striving for the difficult task of near perfect control? Is it worth all the aggravation of harping on your spouse, child, family member or friend if it doesn't make a great deal of difference? Why not lie back and avoid the conflict?

"The Diabetes Control and Complications Trial (DCCT)"

To help answer these questions, the National Institutes of Health initiated a research study in 1983 called the Diabetes Control and Complications Trial (DCCT). In this study, insulin-dependent volunteers between the ages of 13 and 40 with no or minimal early complications were selected from among patients at 21 medical centers throughout the United States and Canada. These patients had been intensively investigated for any evidence of kidney, heart, eye or neurological damage before being selected for the study.

The volunteers were then randomly assigned to two groups. In one, volunteers were treated the way experienced physicians customarily treat patients today: with one or two injections of insulin a day, reasonable diet, exercise, and with insulin dose being adjusted to prevent symptoms of high or low blood sugar. In the second group, intensive efforts were made to achieve perfect control, maintaining blood sugar as close to normal as possible. This was done with the help of an insulin pump (see discussion below on use of the insulin pump) or three or more injections of insulin daily. Diet, exercise, and insulin were evaluated frequently to achieve as close to normal blood sugars as possible. All volunteers made four blood sugar tests per day plus an occasional 3 AM blood test. Both groups were given good medical education and were seen at least four times per year for physical and laboratory checkups.

Conclusive results are in! Intensive control resulted in a 50 to 56 percent reduction in retinopathy, 34 to 56 reduction in proteinuria and kidney damage and 57 to 69% less neuropathy. The study was terminated 2 years early because the results were so conclusive in proving that intensive control dramatically reduces complications.

If you have not already done so, you should speak to your diabetes health caregiver about how you can achieve this level of control: YOUR HEALTHY LIFE MAY LITERALLY DEPEND ON IT.

The Diabetes Control and Complications Trial Conclusions

Conventional Group: 1 or 2 insulin injections daily
Home glucose monitoring
x 1 daily
No daily adjustment of insulin
Visits q 3 month
No telephone contact
No hospitalization to initiate treatment

Intensive Group: 3-4 injections or pump
Home Glucose monitoring 4 or more
times daily
Daily adjustment
Visits every 1 month to the doctor
Frequent telephone contact
Initial hospitalization to start treatment

Goals:

Conventional	Intensive
Avoid symptomatic hyperglycemia	before meal blood sugar 70-120 mgs/%
Maintain growth	1 hr. after meal less 180mg%
Freedom from severe hypoglycemia	3AM blood sugar over 65mg%
	Normal Glycohemoglobin (A_1C)

Results:

1441 patients - in study for 6-5 years
99% completed study
95% scheduled visit
11 died
24 patients to inactive status
8 lost to follow-up

Hemoglobin A_1C's:

44% intensive at one time normal level, whereas the conventional group reached normal in 5%

Retinopathy:

- Primary   -   50% less in intensive group
- Secondary -   Risk of progression reduced by 54% in intensive group compared to conventional
Incidence of severe retinopathy reduced by 47% in intensive
Photocoagulation reduced by 56% in intensive

Nephropathy:
- Primary   -   Microalbuminuria reduced 34% in intensive
                      Macroalbuminuria reduced 44% in intensive
- Secondary -   Microalbuminuria reduced 43% in intensive
                      Macroalbuminuria reduced 56% in intensive

Neuropathy:
- Primary   Reduced   69% in intensive
- Secondary Reduced   57% in intensive

Macrovascular
LDL greater than 160 reduced by 34% in intensive group.

Cardiovascular events reduced by 41% in intensive group.

Severe Hypoglycemia
Three times higher in intensive groups. This is the only major problem that occurred more frequently in the intensive group compared to the conventional group.

- Primary refers to the initial development of a complication. Secondary refers to the worsening of complications once they are there.

Autoimmune Studies

Autoimmunity is a very important topic of interest in diabetes. Autoimmune factors are produced by the body to fight against diseases caused by invasions of bacteria, viruses or foreign substances. They're the reason the healthy body can survive infectious illnesses without antibiotics. But when something goes wrong, the body can't do this, and the ravages of infection can take their toll. That's apparently what happens in AIDS (autoimmune deficiency syndrome). A deficiency of the immune system may account for part of the reason a person with long duration diabetes can be more prone to infection: his immune system has become impaired. However, it may be that an "overactive" or too healthy immune system may be responsible for diabetes developing in the first place.

In addition to fighting disease, particularly infections, the autoimmune system in insulin-dependent people with diabetes backfires and also produces antibodies against the crucial beta cells. Remember, it's the beta cells that produce insulin in the body of a person who does not have diabetes; without those cells, no insulin can be produced. Studies have shown that these antibodies can be present for a number of years before diabetes finally presents itself. Dr. George Eisenbarth and his colleagues at the Joslin Diabetes Center have shown this in their studies with identical twins and triplets; they found that where one sibling had diabetes, the other or others did not.

At Joslin and in other twin studies, it's surprising to find that not all the identical twins develop diabetes. In fact, it's estimated that only 50% of the unaffected Type I twins under the age of 40 will get diabetes like their affected brother or sister. Diabetes will more likely occur if the unaffected twin also has the antibodies against the beta cells. Research must, therefore, answer three questions: Why do the antibodies form in the first place? Do the antibodies against the beta cells cause diabetes? Is there any way of preventing the antibodies from causing the diabetes if the antibodies do develop?

Studies have already been carried out (C.R. Stiller, et al., *Science* 223:1361-1367, 1984) showing that if the immune system can be slowed down in early diabetes by the use of a research drug (cyclosporin A) soon after diabetes is diagnosed, it may reverse the diabetes, and in many cases insulin injections can be stopped. However, restricted diet, good exercise, and the initiation of insulin therapy may be just as effective in reversing the diabetes as cyclosporin A. Before becoming too enthusiastic about drugs such as cyclosporin, remember they have potential side effects and may knock out not only the immune system responsible for the production of the beta cell antibodies, but also those other antibodies necessary for the prevention of cancer and other infections. More studies are needed on these drugs to determine their side effects. Other drugs are being looked into that may prevent the production of beta cell antibodies without knocking off the whole autoimmune system. In other words, a drug could be discovered that will kill off the cells (usually white blood cells) responsible for the production of beta cell antibodies without killing off other important cells that produce antibodies that protect the body from infections and possibly cancer.

Other places where research is needed in order to determine the role autoimmunity plays in diabetes include those implicating a possible viral cause, and in studies connected with beta cell and pancreatic transplantation. Here finding a way to prevent rejection of transplanted pancreas would be very insightful.

Viruses

In the forefront of diabetes research is the difficult task of discovering whether or not viruses are a possible cause of diabetes, especially the type I insulin-dependent diabetes. Mumps is one of the viruses commonly suspected as a possible cause of diabetes. Over the past 100 years, there have been many medical reports of patients who developed diabetes shortly after a mumps illness as well as reports on increased incidence of diabetes in the general population occurring after a mumps epidemic. In one medical journal, there was a report of a 10-month-old baby who did not have any of the usual characteristics of mumps but who did have two brothers who had had mumps shortly before the baby was diagnosed with diabetes. The baby's doctors then performed blood tests to see whether or not the blood contained antibodies to mumps. Sure enough, antibodies were found.

This case is a good example of why it is so hard to implicate viruses. Viral diseases can be manifested by minimal symptoms or by so few typical ones that the diagnosis is obscured. It is not uncommon for a patient diagnosed with sudden onset diabetes to have no recall of a previous illness that may in fact have triggered the diabetes.

In my own practice, I have often suspected that a viral factor is responsible for the onset of diabetes. In one particular family with no previous history of diabetes, two brothers and a sister all developed insulin-dependent diabetes; these siblings were all under the age of 10, and they all had had mumps at various times before the onset of the diabetes. Although this information is suggestive, it is by no means conclusive when we consider that mumps had affected over 90% of the population, at least until the mumps vaccine became available.

Besides the mumps virus, numerous other viruses have been implicated as a cause for diabetes. These include hepatitis viruses, infectious mononucleosis virus, German measles virus, influenza virus (it was the influenza of 1968 that triggered my own diabetes; one day I was perfectly fine, the next day I had intense symptoms of diabetes along with symptoms of influenza), the common cold viruses, and more recently, a virus called Coxsackie B4 virus.

Other factors indicating the possible role of viruses include the following:

- There seem to be seasonal peaks when diabetes occurs, corresponding to the times these viruses are most active
- Diabetes frequently occurs in patients who have no family history of the disease
- Inflammatory cells (which occur in response to a viral attack) are frequently found in the pancreas (where the beta cells are located) in patients with diabetes
- Antibodies to the beta cells are frequently found in insulin dependent diabetes. Regarding this last point, people normally don't have antibodies to their own cells; thus, they shouldn't have antibodies to beta cells. However, if a virus attacks the beta cells or injures them, the beta cells could possibly act like foreign cells, causing the formation of beta cell antibodies, resulting in diabetes.

Researchers Dr. John Craighead in Vermont and Dr. Abner L. Notkins at the National Institutes of Health have done extensive research on viruses and have demonstrated the development of diabetes by injecting mice with various viruses. When the pancreata of the mice were studied, there was microscopic evidence that the viruses affected the beta cells.

The most convincing case of a virus being the cause of human diabetes occurred in 1978, when a young boy died with newly onset diabetes. At postmortem the doctors found damage to the beta cells. They then isolated from the pancreas a virus similar to the Coxsackie B4, grew the virus, and then injected it into mice. Some of the mice then developed diabetes. Although the case seems fairly conclusive, there is room for doubt since an estimated 40% of adults have antibodies to the Coxsackie B4 virus, yet the number of people who develop diabetes is much less.

However, if it can be concluded that some forms of insulin-dependent diabetes are caused by a virus or viruses, then it is possible that a vaccine can be made that could make these types of diabetes as easily prevent able as polio, small-pox, and other viral or infectious diseases.

Insulin

Considerable research is being done on insulin itself. As discussed earlier in Chapter 9, "Insulin: A Miracle Medicine," we have come a long way in purifying insulin. Some of the insulin that is used today comes from the pancreata of cattle and swine. These insulins originally contained many impurities. Over the years, most of the impurities have been eliminated so that animal insulins now used are over 99% pure insulins.

Problems remain, however, with respect to the use of insulin from cattle and swine. Although these insulins are essentially purified, the insulin itself is slightly different in structure from human insulin. As you recall, insulin is a protein and is made up of approximately 51 amino acids. Pork insulin has 1 amino acid that is different from human insulin. Beef insulin has 3 amino acids that are different from human insulin. Thus, with the slight impurity and the slight variation of the presently available animal insulins, there is still the possibility of insulin allergy or insulin resistance (requiring large amounts of insulin to overcome the anti-insulin antibodies that the body produces?

Great advances have been made in overcoming the allergy and insulin resistance associated with pork and beef insulins by the actual production of human insulin.

Bacterially-Produced and Recombinant DNA Human Insulin

Production of human insulin through the aid of bacteria may prove to be a more significant advancement. In late 1978, Genentech, a California-based company, developed a technique for producing human insulin through its genetic engineering research In this technique, the human insulin gene or the gene components that control insulin production are synthesized in the laboratory. The synthesized gene components are then inserted into the DNA (genetic material) of the bacteria called *E. coli*. As the bacteria multiply, they generate the human insulin components, which can then be extracted and combined.

The Eli Lilly Company, which is the largest manufacturer of insulin in the United States, now uses Genentech's techniques to produce human insulin in their Humulin products.

Recombinant DNA human insulin is now being produced by Novo-Nordisk Company, the Hoechst Company, pharmaceutical leaders in the diabetes field.The recombinant DNA Human Insulins have shown a decrease in the incidence of insulin allergy and insulin resistance. Furthermore, we now have unlimited source of insulin by these methods, which could make insulin much less expensive and eliminate the need for animal insulins that are still being used.

Faster Acting Regular Insulin

Eli Lilly has developed a new insulin analog called *Lys-Pro* or Humalog, which has been shown to have a faster onset of action after subcutaneous injection. This insulin may be better than Regular insulin for two good reasons:

- It may peak in the blood stream very quickly, so that high levels of insulin will prevent the high blood sugars that occur after eating, especially heavy carbohydrate meals. This may be similar to what happens after a non-diabetic person eats where the insulin rapidly comes out of the pancreatic beta cells to keep the blood sugar normal. Presently the Regular Insulin we are using does not peak until 1 to 3 hours after injection, so that blood sugars are frequently very high 1 to 2 hours after eating.
- The new Lispro or Humalog Human insulin is disposed of more quickly so that only small amounts of it remain after 4 to 5 hours. This may be helpful in preventing the hypoglycemia (or low blood sugars) that occur could possibly occur with Regular insulin. It may be useful in very young children who are not eating well - then insulin can be adjusted and given during the meal depending on the amount they've eaten.

So better control and less hypoglycemia is the hope. Eli Lilly has been working on research studies that have substantiated this.

Insulin Pumps

Some people with diabetes, especially those who have had the disease for a long time, have brittle diabetes, in which good control is virtually impossible because blood sugars fluctuate markedly with only minimal changes in food intake, insulin dose or physical activity. Also, there is an increased tendency toward low blood sugar or high blood sugar coma.

Unable to achieve good control, patients may be more susceptible to some of the chronic complications. Doctors have been baffled by the phenomenon of brittle diabetes, wondering whether patients were"cheating" on their diet, skipping meals of insulin doses, or whether their emotional state was having an adverse effect on control. However, even when these patients are hospitalized under controlled conditions, it is difficult to get perfect control despite good diet and frequent blood sugar monitoring (as you'll remember from my discussion in Chapter 11, "The Effects of Insulin Over-Use; Brittle Diabetes and the Somoygi Effects").

Technological advances have introduced the possibility of managing this type of diabetes with the use of a portable infusion pump. There are several types of insulin pumps, all geared to deliver a steady amount of regular insulin every few minutes at a basal rate, so that over a 24-hour period approximately 15 to 30 units of regular insulin have been delivered. In addition, approximately 20 to 30 minutes before each major meal and heavy snacks an additional amount of regular insulin (generally between 2 and 10 units) can be injected or "bolused."

Some of the results of research studies from around the world have used insulin pumps, such as that used in the Diabetes Control and Complications Trial (DCCT). The following describes the use of the pump in a young man with diabetes that had been nearly impossible to control.

Man Helped by Pump

This case involved a middle-aged man, who had had diabetes since he was a teenager. When it was first diagnosed, he had difficulty controlling blood sugars and even had an episode of ketoacidosis. As he got older, he could prevent episodes of ketoacidosis and extremely high blood sugars, but blood sugars still bounced around excessively despite proper diet and regular exercise. In addition, he was prone to hypoglycemic episodes, some of which were quite severe.

With this history, we brought him into the hospital hoping to achieve better control. His prehospital insulin dose was 34 NPH, 6 regular before breakfast and 6 NPH, 4 regular before supper. See hospital daily blood sugar and insulin log showing this man's daily blood sugar levels and insulin dose (he was put on a diet of approximately 1800 calories) on the pages following this discussion. As the table indicates, we were hoping to get good control during this hospitalization with regular insulin before each main meal, along with intermediate-acting insulin NPH in the morning and before supper (refer to the table listing results during the first hospitalization).

At this point, the patient had had enough (due to his lack of improvement) and discharged himself from the hospital.

Approximately six weeks later, we readmitted him in another effort to see if we could establish control with the help of an insulin pump. (see the table showing results during the second hospitalization).

This time the patient was tremendously pleased with his progress, and the doctor discharged him from the hospital.

It should be noted that on the readmission date of April 11 his blood sugar was 518mg%, and blood sugars remained well out of control until April 15. The insulin pump was then started. The blood sugars that followed over the next four days were the best consecutive blood sugars that this man had ever had. I saw him in a follow-up office visit several days later with a blood sugar of 84mg%, the first normal blood sugar he had had in the office in 10 consecutive office visits! In addition, his glycohemoglobin level, an index of diabetes control, fell from 10.9% (poor control) to 7.9%, which is in the normal range.

First Hospitalization Without Insulin Pump

Date	Blood Sugars (mg)	Time	Insulin Dose (in units)	When Dose Was Given
February 13	357	Fasting	26 NPH	Before
	or 7 AM		6 Regular	Breakfast
	–	11 AM		
	255	3 PM	4 Regular	Before
				Supper
February 14	125	7 AM	12 NPH	Before
			10 Regular	Breakfast
	361	11 AM	4 Regular	Before Lunch
	248	3 PM	6 Regular	Before
				Supper
February 15	506	7 AM	12 NPH	Before
			10 Regular	Breakfast
	550	11 AM	4 Regular	Before Lunch
	356	3 PM	6 NPH	Before
			6 Regular	Supper
February 16	386	7 AM	12NPH	Before
			10 regular	Breakfast
	453	11 AM	6 Regular	Before Lunch
	188	3 PM	4 NPH	Before
			4 Regular	Supper
February 17	419	7 AM	8 NPH	Before
			6 Regular	Breakfast
	513	11 AM	4 Regular	Before Lunch
	322	3 PM	8 NPH	Before
			6 Regular	Supper
February 18	564	7 AM	14 NPH	Before
			14 Regular	Breakfast
	570	11 AM	8 regular	Before Lunch
	304	3 PM	8 NPH	Before
			6 Regular	Supper
February 19	549	7 AM	20 NPH	Before
			10 Regular	Breakfast
	543	11 AM	4 regular	Before Lunch
	213	3 PM	4 NPH	Before
			4 Regular	Supper
		9 PM	4 NPH 4 regular	Before Bed
February 20	480	7 AM	32 NPH	Before
			6 regular	Breakfast
	500	11 AM	18 regular	Before Lunch
	96	3 PM	6 NPH	Before Supper

Second Hospitalization Before Pump Started

Date	Blood Sugars (mg)	Time	Insulin Dose (in units)	When Dose Was Given
April 11		7 AM	36 NPH	Before
			4 Regular	Breakfast
		11 AM		
	518	3 PM	6 NPH	Before
			4 Regular	Supper
		9 PM		
April 12	123	7 AM	36 NPH	Before
			6 Regular	Breakfast
	302	11 AM		
	179	3 PM	4 NPH	Before
			4 Regular	Supper
		9 PM		
April 13	397	7 AM	20 NPH	Before
			10 Regular	Breakfast
		11 AM	15 Regular	Before Lunch
	402	3 PM	8 NPH	Before
			8 Regular	Supper
	202	9 PM		
April 14	604	7 AM	20 NPH	Before
			10 Regular	Breakfast
	590	11 AM	15 Regular	Before Lunch
	307	3 PM	Pump Started	

After Pump Started (Basal Rate: 26 reg/24 hrs)

Date	Blood Sugars (mg)	Time	Insulin Dose (in units)	When Dose Was Given
April 15	77	7 AM	9 Regular	Before Breakfast
	160	11 AM	3 Regular	Before Lunch
	156	3 PM	6 Regular	Before Supper
	105	9 PM	3 Regular	Before Night Snack
April 16	177	7 AM	9 Regular	Before Breakfast
	247	11 AM	3 Regular	Before Lunch
	203	3 PM	6 Regular	Before Supper
	177	9 PM	6 Regular	Before Night Snack
April 17	53	7 AM	9 Regular	Before Breakfast
	141	11 AM	3 Regular	Before Lunch
	117	3 PM	6 Regular	Before Supper
	97	9 PM	6 Regular	Before Night Snack
April 18	64	7 AM	9 Regular	Before Breakfast

The use of portable pumps is an exciting and encouraging regimen of treatment for trying to get better control. However, it should be emphasized that these pumps are not necessarily appropriate for everyone with diabetes; there are some potential drawbacks. As they appear now, the pumps have to be worn on a belt, shoulder holster or the pouch of a garment. The site of injection is subcutaneous, as in an insulin injection, and the site has to be changed every two to four days. Patients feel "wired" to them as the insulin has to be given through a tubing from the pump. This may disrupt sexual activity for some people, although the better control may make even better as they are more primed for it. In addition, pumps may interfere with some other forms of recreation, particularly swimming, since some of the pumps are not waterproof. In such a case, the patient must detach the pump from the tubing while he swims and reattach it after the swim.

Another problem that patients should be aware of is that the pump may need "reprogramming" every so often. That is, there are times when more or less insulin may be needed. For instance, if you refer to the man just described, you can see he was programmed to get 26 units regular insulin basal rate, 6 regular before breakfast, 6 regular before lunch, 6 regular before supper, and 6 regular before the night snack. If this man gets ill or overeats, he may need to take some extra insulin to get his blood sugars back to normal; if he overexercises, he may need slightly less insulin. Thus, at this stage in insulin pump development, it is obvious that these pumps are quite demanding.

But for those users who are satisfied with their improved diabetes control and the resulting sense of well-being, the inconvenience and demands of the pump seem a minimal trade-off. Many patients do not want to be without them until better therapy is available.

Potential Improvements in the Insulin Pump

Further improvements on the insulin pump will focus on making them smaller and therefore easier to carry or wear.

Progress is also being made in the design of an implantable insulin pump, which would make this device even more convenient. However, implanted pumps would not be as accessible. Insulin would still have to be injected into the pumps, and they would have to have a remote control program to adjust them when more or less insulin was needed, or to stop them in case of malfunction.

Another major ideal feature would be the development of a glucose sensor. Ideally, this sensor would constantly measure the blood sugar level and then relay a message to the insulin pump to discharge automatically more or less insulin in order to keep blood sugars in the normal range. The combined unit would in fact be an artificial beta cell, in that it would automatically adjust insulin in response to blood sugar levels.

Although this artificial beta cell sounds simple enough, it is quite a complicated thing to develop. Scientists have been working on the development of this glucose sensor for over 25 years now, and millions of dollars have been spent without major success. Yet the prospects are brightening. Apparently, the greatest obstacle in the development of an implantable glucose sensor is making it compatible with human tissues. Just as the human body may reject a transplanted heart or kidney, it may also reject the glucose sensor. Researchers at centers such as the Joslin Diabetes Center in Boston are hopeful that this rejection process can be overcome.

If this artificial beta cell becomes available, it would be superior to the portable insulin pump since it would allow for variations in food intake and automatically make adjustments in insulin dose to keep the blood sugar normal. Problems that remain to be solved include where in the body to place the insulin pump, how to get the insulin into the pump, and how to make sure the pump is working correctly.

The Doctor Tries the NovoPen

It has now been over 28 years since I developed diabetes. Wanting to have experienced the insulin pump myself to see what improved control I could get, so that I may best counsel and instruct my patients on the pro's and con's of the computerized automatic insulin pumps, I tried the insulin pump myself. In fact, I was able to obtain a glycohemoglobin level in the 6.1% range (similar to that obtained by some of my more outstanding patients). On the unfavorable side, it was a bit of a nuisance for me (although not for many of my patients). It inhibited me from literally "jumping into

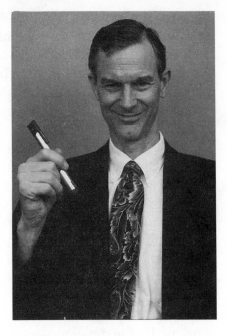

the lake" (that is, when I go on vacation) or the Jacuzzi. Also, I've been on a doctors' research study with aspirin to see if aspirin prevents heart attacks. (As you can see, I enjoy research studies.) This has caused pain and bleeding at the insulin pump infusion site especially when I am about to crush an overhead tennis shot or to drive one of my wicked forehands passed an opponent.

The answers to this dilemma came with the arrival in 1986 of the NovoPen® (Novo-Nordisk) and its successor the NovoPen® 1.5. A nifty device the size of a pen, it allows me to always have regular insulin available in my pen pocket to allow me to bolus regular insulin just before mealtimes (at the hospital, lake, restaurant or tennis court) in a very inconspicuous manner. To get my basal insulin I take Lente insulin in the evening to keep my fasting blood sugars down. The success I've had is reflected in my last three glycohemoglobins of 6.9%, 7.4% and 8.5%. The NovoPen® 1.5 device is very economical compared to the very expensive computerized pumps, and I would definitely recommend it for those interested in getting the best control possible with the help of the

Bolus-Basal insulin technique as discussed in this chapter and the insulin chapter. NovoNordisk also makes Novolin Prefilled™, a disposable insulin pen with the ability to deliver up to 58 units of insulin in a single dose. Novolin Prefilled™ comes filled with 150 units of N, R, or 70/30 Novolin Human Insulin.

Pancreas or Beta Cell Transplantation

The above techniques offer encouraging possibilities in the effective treatment of diabetes through artificial devices. What about live techniques such as transplantation of healthy insulin-secreting cells into patients with diabetes? Research into these possibilities has been going on for over 30 years with the hope that this will lead to successful transplantation of either the whole pancreas or only the insulin-secreting beta cells. It has already been demonstrated in experimental animals with diabetes that it can be reversed at least temporarily, with either of these procedures. Even more encouraging is the fact that by reversing diabetes with these techniques, some of the diabetes complications that occur in these animals can be prevented, delayed, or even reversed with the use of transplants.

Theoretically, transplantation seems simple enough, but there are major problems. Transplantation of the whole pancreas is a risky operation. Infections, heart attacks, and the destruction of pancreatic tissue are serious life-threatening situations that would need to be addressed directly after surgery. Then there is the problem of pancreas rejection. The rejection process occurs because of the normal body's immune system, which produces white blood cells and antibodies to the transplanted tissues. The only time that rejection would not occur is when the donated transplanted tissue is nearly identical to the recipient's tissue. In all other cases, large doses of powerful medication would be necessary to counteract this rejection phenomenon. These medicines have serious side effects, some of which make patients very prone to infection. Considering the problems involved, it is clear why transplantation of the pancreas has not been performed often. In most cases of pancreas transplantation, the diabetes was complicated by life-threatening processes due to the many risks associated with the transplantation surgery. In some cases, there was considerable improvement in the control of the diabetes, but unfortunately, the extended life span of these patients was less than two years.

Research is being done on the beta or islet cells themselves. It has been estimated that it only takes one ounce or less of beta cells to produce the desired insulin to control diabetes. Again, animal studies have been very encouraging, showing the reversibility of the diabetes. The operation is much simpler than transplanting the whole pancreas.

The problem remains, however, of how to procure enough of the beta or islet cells. The cells must come from the pancreas. In isolating the cells, much of the pancreas has to be destroyed as well. Once the cells are isolated, they must be preserved. Research is being done on how to obtain a greater quantity of cells.

As described in a recent issue of Diabetes Interview, Dr. Barry Solomon Ph.D. has been working to develop techniques of harvesting pig islet cells. There are up to 80 million pigs slaughtered for food every year. This means the availability of 80 million pig pancreases. The beta cells from these islets can be isolated and made available for transplantation.

The problem then remains: How to prevent the body's immune rejection process. As in the case of pancreatic transplantation patients, large doses of medication with potentially dangerous side effects could be used to prevent the rejection process. Better still would be a way of avoiding the use of these medications.

Researchers, working with Dr. Soloman, have taken the isolated pig islet or beta cells and placed them in the hockey puck sized device that can be placed in the patient's abdomen. The device is then attached to a vein to keep blood flowing thought it. The beta cells are protected from the immune system in a plastic membrane. The beta cells can sense the body's blood sugar level, make and release insulin and stop insulin when the blood sugar is getting low. In addition the membrane is permeable to oxygen, glucose and other nutrients to help keep the beta cells thriving.

As there are procedures being worked on there is continued research being done to find drugs that will prevent the immune rejection process without as many side effects.

Research on Type II Diabetes

Much of this discussion centers on Type I insulin-treated diabetes. But what about Type II non-insulin-dependent diabetes (which is by far the most common type)? Here too, much information has been accumulated over the last several years, which may generate some answers. As discussed in earlier chapters, it has been found that 80% of Type II non-insulin-treated people actually have elevated blood insulin levels. Theoretically, the high blood insulin should keep blood sugar levels normal or even low, especially if the insulin levels are higher than normal. But for some reason, the body cells resist the effect of insulin in Type II diabetes.

Normally, body cells have "receptors" that receive insulin so that it can keep blood glucose levels within a normal range. In the non-insulin-dependent adult with diabetes, it is thought that these receptors do not function properly or that there are not enough of them. When this happens, diabetes develops despite high insulin levels. In addition, the high insulin levels may contribute to obesity, which further complicates the diabetes. Obesity, lack of exercise, and overeating may all contribute to the receptor defect. The latest oral medications that overcome this defect may be forthcoming. There are also studies with medications such as Miglitol and Acarbose that work in the intestinal tract to slow down the absorption of sugar and thereby prevent the high blood sugar that occurs after eating. These may be effective in both Type I and Type II diabetes. Metformin (Glucophage) as previously been discussed in the pill chapter, can definitely reduce the amount of insulin needed injection to control blood sugar. Finally, Troglitazone is another class of insulin sensitizing agents which may improve the body cells' ability to use sugar. These agents may have the duality of lowering blood sugar and possibly the body cholesterol as well.

Some insight into treatment of non-insulin-dependent diabetes may also be found in research work with Glucagon. As indicated in earlier chapters, Glucagon is a substance which, like insulin, is produced by the islet cells of the pancreas. However, it has the opposite effect from insulin raises blood sugar. Might the over production of Glucagon be implicated in the development of diabetes? Most researchers think not, but efforts are being made to explore further this obvious possibility.

Glucagon also contributes to diabetes coma with ketoacidosis. There are some Type I peoples with diabetes who are particularly prone to this type of coma. It has been shown that if glucagon blood levels can be suppressed, there will be less risk of ketoacidosis. Work is presently being done with a substance called Somatostatin, the third substance (in addition to Glucagon and Insulin) produced by the islet cells of the pancreas. Somatostatin has been shown to decrease Glucagon levels and delay the onset of ketoacidosis in animals with diabetes when insulin is withheld. Somatostatin may have the same effect on humans. It remains to be proven, however, that Somatostatin will have no serious side effects, and its effect must extend beyond just a few hours. At present, Somatostatin must be given by injection, and this means the inconvenience of several injections per day.

Research on Diabetes Complications

What about some of the complications of diabetes? Have there been any advances in their treatment? With regard to eye complications, use of the laser beam has been successful in avoiding permanent loss of vision. However, it is essential to diagnose eye problems while they are in their earliest stages. It is also important to realize that severe Retinopathy may be present without any visual impairment to alert the person with diabetes that loss of vision may soon occur.

That's why it is of the utmost importance for people with diabetes to have frequent eye examinations by physicians who are familiar with diabetes Retinopathy.

New computerized fiber optic technology is being developed at The Joslin Vision Network which will help diagnose retinopathy instantly when the patient is at the eye doctor's office. This will allow medical investigators to determine the efficacy of new drugs and therapies in months instead of years.

Impotence is another very frequent complication of diabetes. Recent studies indicate that impotence may be caused by damage to either nerves or blood vessels (arteriosclerosis) that supply the penis. It is not unusual for impotence to be the initial symptom leading to the diagnosis of diabetes, although current thinking is that diabetes is present for a considerable time before this symptom presents itself. It is possible that good control of the diabetes will relieve this symptom, but in cases where the nervous system or vascular system has been severely affected, it may be too late. (This is one more reason why early diagnosis of diabetes is important, so that treatment can be given as soon as possible.) Some success has been shown in recent work on blood vessels to improve the blood supply to the penis. Studies with male hormone therapy have shown no improvement in performance, although this type of therapy may stimulate sexual desire, which is doubly frustrating under these conditions. Moderate success has been achieved through surgical penile implants, which allow good performance during intercourse, penile injections and improved vacuum devices. New topical penile creams may prove effective in improving sexual functions.

An additional complication that may plague the person with diabetes is neuritis, resulting from inflammation and disease of the nerves. It can cause extreme pain that can become unbearable, with associated sleepless nights, depression, and irritability. Numerous medicines have been used to control the pain, but the medicines (Amitriptyline and Fluphenazine) have been proven to be somewhat effective. However, these medications themselves may have adverse side effects. A Nerve Growth Factor is being studied hoping that it will help regrow damaged nerves to relieve the pain from this condition.

Vitamins remain a possible therapeutic modality that may prevent some of the complications - as discussed earlier. Vitamin C, 1000 mg; vitamin E, 400 I.U., Selenium, Magnesium and other vitamins may all be needed. I personally have been using JuicePlus, complex capsules containing many of these natural vitamins, phytonutrients, and minerals hoping they may cut down on the vascular complication which vegetarians seem to have less of.

Folic Acid of 1 mg or more may also be effective in reducing the concentrations of Homocysteine. Homocysteine is converted from methionine found in many foods. Taking folic acid may help prevent the conversion of methionine to Homocysteine in the body. Patients on folic acid have shown a reduced Homocysteine level as reported in the *Journal of American Medical Association*, 1995 Vol. 274 (13) 1049-1057.

Other Biomedical Research Studies

Since high blood sugar may be the culprit in the early complications; of diabetes, and since it is practically impossible to keep blood sugar normal all of the time for most people with diabetes (the person most motivated to achieve this is a woman who is pregnant), studies are being done in many centers to see if, even allowing for high blood sugars, the complications that result from them can be prevented. More simply, since we can't prevent high blood sugar in most people with diabetes all the time (overeating, lack of insulin or exercise), then possibly we can prevent the complication by preventing the high blood sugar from doing its damage.

One of the ways high blood sugar is thought to cause the complications of Cataracts, Retinopathy, and Neuropathy is through the conversion of the extra sugar (glucose) into Sorbitol (another sugar form that is sometimes used to sweeten candies) by the enzyme aldose reductase. This occurs inside the lens of the eye, the retina, or the nerve cells. The accumulation of sorbitol inside the cells somehow causes the damage. Scientists at the National Institutes of Health and other places have been working on inhibitors of Aldose Reductase, such as Sorbinil and Tolrestat, in an effort to prevent the accumulation of sorbitol that occurs from the conversion of blood glucose. So far, studies with these Aldose Reductase inhibitor agents have shown some good results in preventing and reversing cataracts and neuropathy in animals. Now studies are being done with their human counterparts, hoping to find similar good results without adverse side effects.

Another way Aldose Reductase and high blood sugar may cause damage is by somehow decreasing accumulation of Myoinositol (an ingredient you will find in some vitamin preparations). Apparently high blood sugar and high sorbitol levels affect the ability of some cells to take up and store myoinositol. In nerve tissue particularly, lack of Myoinositol causes an effect on nerve function and, because of this, eventual neuropathy. Some studies indicate that with adequate oral supplements of inositol (300-to-900mg) the cells may be able to get sufficient quantities of Myoinositol, even in the face of high blood sugar.

Two other ways high blood sugar or glucose attack is by combining with various body proteins. This is exemplified particularly by the glycohemoglobin, as discussed in Chapter 12, "One of the Latest Tests: Measurement of Glycohemoglobin." As a reminder, hemoglobin is found within red blood cells, which live for three to four months inside the blood circulatory system. Hemoglobin's job is to carry oxygen to the tissue and then remove carbon dioxide to the lungs. As hemoglobin is doing its job, it comes in contact with blood sugar or glucose. The poorer the diabetes control, the higher the glucose in the blood and therefore the more glucose that can combine with hemoglobin to form glycohemoglobin. Glycohemoglobin apparently does not do as good a job as hemoglobin in carrying on its basic function of oxygen and carbon dioxide delivery. Also, as glucose can combine with hemoglobin, it maybe combined with many other proteins— particularly the lining of blood vessels, thereby interferring with blood vessels functioning especially in the kidney for instance an so may be responsible for some of the long term vascular complications of diabetes, and thereby cause part of the vascular complications of long-term diabetes.

By now, it should be evident that while there is a tremendous amount still to be learned about diabetes, much has been accomplished. What we know about diabetes developed from work done hundreds of years ago by physicians and scientists who struggled to lay the ground work for future research efforts. In medical research, steps can only be taken one at a time, and each step is very costly in terms of the money and time involved. It takes dedication and sacrifice on the part of the researchers, who give up the very considerable monetary rewards they could achieve in other fields. It is important that the public support the research efforts of these dedicated people. Both emotional and financial backing is needed so that researchers will not become frustrated at the slow rate of progress. Through the many diabetes associations, public support can sustain the morale of the researchers and the momentum of their efforts as they strive to find answers in solving problems of diabetes.

31

The Ten Most Asked Questions

Their Answers

Do you ever overeat or indulge in sweets? This is a
favorite question with my patients, and there are several ways
I can answer it. I can plead the Fifth Amendment, refusing to
answer for fear that my answer might incriminate me, or I can
refer you back to (Chapter 18, "The Glycemic Index and the
Sweet Tooth." But to be more straightforward, you may occasionally find me, like my fellow human beings, lapsing into
an occasional indulgence or eating more than my diet allows.
The fact is that it's very hard, nearly impossible, not to give in
to the insuppressible appetite that people with diabetes have.
In my treatment of more than 8,000 people with diabetes, I
know hardly one of them, including myself, who's been 100%
perfect with his or her diet—hunger is always there.

I would bet that even such a great man as Nathan Pritikin,
as you know he pleaded with people to follow a very restricted diet, would have a hard time if he had diabetes and had to
restrict his Pritikin foods to keep his blood sugar controlled.
A comparison that I think amplifies the predicament of the
person with diabetes even further is a comparison with the
smoker or the alcohol drinker. If the smoker or the drinker
does not take the first smoke or the first drink, he can fare
pretty well. It's a matter of not having the first smoke or first
drink. But with diabetes, it's not so simple. Food is necessary
for survival. Once you take the first bite, it's hard to stop at
the limited amount necessary to control weight and blood
sugar—whether it's a peanut butter sandwich or ice cream.
So, to answer the original question, yes, I do occasionally slip
up and eat sweets or overindulge, but my awareness of the

crucial importance of good control keeps me from doing it often.

Can insulin be taken through the nose? Patients are always looking for an easier way of giving insulin than by the "needle." It can't be given by mouth because it's destroyed by the processes of digestion. It can be given by subcutaneous insulin pumps, where insulin is delivered under the skin. As discussed in the research chapter, insulin pumps are not the easiest to use.

Hoping to find an easier way of giving insulin, investigators have attempted to give insulin by a nasal spray (*New England Journal of Medicine* 3 12; 1088,1985). This was done over a three-month period, and the researchers were happy with their results in lowering blood sugars after meals. However, they also indicated several thorny problems such as cost, the need for a very concentrated U-500 insulin, and the fact that the insulin only lasted four hours, so that a separate injection still had to be given to achieve insulin effect throughout the night. In addition, the investigators were concerned that the nasal irritation associated with colds or sinus infections might be a potential problem. Further investigation is continuing to see whether these problems can be resolved. It is also possible that instead of a nasal spray, insulin preparations will be made that can be absorbed through the skin or the eyes (in the form of eye drops).

How is it possible that many people with diabetes go undiagnosed? Many people with diabetes go undiagnosed because an elevated blood sugar may not cause a person to feel sick. Despite feeling well, vascular disease may progress until a major medical problem occurs, i.e., heart attack, impotence, neuritis.

You discuss being one's own doctor—what does that mean? Diet, exercise, insulin, stress, emotion and travel are a few of the factors that affect the control of blood sugar. Since we're all unique, these factors affect each person differently.

Even if a physician sees a patient regularly, these effects are difficult to determine. Consequently, the patient needs to evaluate his or her own symptoms and, in a sense, assume the role of being his or her own doctor. Learn as much about diabetes as possible, test blood sugars frequently and learn how to prevent problems of diabetes.

What helps a person keep his diabetes controlled? Goals, goals, goals. I believe that setting goals is crucial to keeping diabetes controlled. But first the person with diabetes must realize that it's important to keep diabetes controlled. Some people with diabetes, and even some doctors and nurses, have their doubts about the degree of control people with diabetes need to get, but everyone agrees that good control is crucial.

One man I spoke with recently, adamantly refused to listen to my recommendations about the value of good control, as he puffed away on a pack of cigarettes. He said, "Prove to me that good control will extend my life 20 years, and I'll do what you suggest." With that attitude and with the fact that he felt well, he wasn't about to listen. However, even for those who see the value of good control, many still have a tough time achieving it. This is because so many people with diabetes feel reasonably well, despite high blood sugars, so they put off their attempts to diet or test blood sugar or exercise saying, "I'll start tomorrow." The problem is that "tomorrow" never comes, and the diabetes can progress unchecked.

To avoid this natural human tendency to delay, setting goals helps. Set reasonable goals, though, not outlandish ones. Most people are competitive, at least in the sense that they get satisfaction from achieving their goals. For the person who wants to lose weight, set. a goal of one half to four pounds per month. Enlist the aid of Weight Watchers, LeanLine, or Overeaters Anonymous, if that's necessary to help achieve the goal. Weight checks every week will help, too. Cut back on the carbohydrates, also.

To help achieve good diabetes control, set goals for the blood sugar levels you would like to attain. Ideally, you should aim for levels of 70 to 140mg% premeals and 100 to 160mg% after eating. By setting these blood sugar goals, it is incentive to do the tests that will help you analyze the factors that affect control, such as diet, exercise, insulin, and stressful environmental factors, then make the appropriate changes in those areas to ensure that you reach the goals you set. Finally, it's also important to set goals when you are exercising. It's not too common for a person to come home from work dog-tired, and decide it's time to get up and run a few miles or get on the rowing machine. More likely, such a person will put it off until tomorrow However, if you set a goal of half a mile per day or five miles per week, it will stir your competitive spirit to achieve these goals and then go for higher ones.

It's important to reward and affirm yourself after acheiving your obtainable goals. Buy that book you've been wanting to read, take in a movie and yes, ladies why not buy that dress you've been waiting to go on sale! Celebrate, you've earned it.

Since many people with diabetes go undiagnosed, and a typical complication of diabetes is impotence, is it possible that many impotent men have diabetes and that with proper diagnosis and treatment their impotence should be secured? Yes, as I discussed in Chapter 24, "Men and Diabetes: Sexual Dysfunction", up to 50% of the male diabetes population is impotent. Impotence results from complications of the nervous and vascular systems. I believe that early detection and good control of diabetes can prevent impotence.

You are a tennis champion and a runner. How has diabetes affected your athletic endeavors? Yes, I have been the champion of my club and have won outside tournaments as well. Due to careful control, my diabetes has not affected my athletic pursuits, although I do experience transient hypoglycemic episodes. My strength, coordination, speed, and athletic ability are as good as any 50-year-old's, and perhaps better than many 25-year-old's.

How often should the blood sugar be tested? Depending on what type of diabetes the person has (insulin- or non-insulin-dependent), the stage of diabetes, the degree of control a person is striving for, as well as other associated conditions such as pregnancy or illness, it can be tested anywhere from one-to-two times a week up to four-to-six times a day. For anyone with diabetes, blood sugar testing can be self-educational. It demonstrates the response of the blood sugar to various factors such as illness, stress, food, exercise. So when a person first finds out that he has diabetes, the more he tests the more he'll learn of these interrelationships.

However, once he discovers these interrelationships and he's satisfied with his control (especially if blood sugar is normal at 60 to 120mg% and he has non-insulin-dependent diabetes), he may cut his testing back to one-to-two times a week, performing the tests after eating. As long as the blood sugar stays under 140mg%, all is well. However, if it starts going higher, more frequent testing is in order.

For an insulin-dependent person aiming for as good control as possible, tests should be done before each meal and at bell until blood sugar levels are satisfactory. Ideally, they should fall between 80mg% and 140mg%. However, for some the goal may not have to be quite so good (for instance an older person). Once the pre-meal blood sugar is satisfactory, a person may want to test his blood sugars after meals to keep them between 100mg% and 180mg%. Once all these blood sugars are consistent and satisfactory, it may be all right to cut back the frequency of testing to just five or six times per week at varying times of the day. If the blood sugar tests start going higher, more frequent testing is again in order. More blood sugar testing is also recommended during periods of illness, during pregnancy, and to help prevent high and low blood sugar reactions as discussed else where in this book.

How do I get my diabetes under control when I'm taking my insulin and getting plenty of exercise? You should find out what is causing your blood sugars to be running so high and then figure out what to do to improve them. I would advise, as Dr. Richard Bernstein did 28 years ago, testing your blood sugars seven to ten times a day. You may then find out some surprising things. I can't generalize because for each person with diabetes there are individual differences. You may find that so-called "diabetic foods" or complex carbohydrates can cause just as much of a rise in blood sugar as sweets. In my long experience with over 10,000 people with diabetes, over-consumption of bread, crackers, milk, juice and other "innocent" carbohydrates can wreak just as much havoc to diabetes control as sweets. You must realize that a blood sugar of 100 is equivalent to one teaspoon of sugar (or five grams) in the bloodstream. Since one "bread exchange" has 15 grams of carbohydrates, which are rapidly converted to sugar in the bloodstream, you can see how a few extra crackers or extra bread can mean the difference between a blood sugar of 40 or one over 200.

Keep testing your blood sugar and work with your nutritionist or doctor to see if appropriate dietary changes, insulin changes, exercise changes or stress changes can improve your control. These are just a few of the things I would suggest to start you off.

Is diabetes hereditary? Understanding the hereditary aspects of diabetes presents a real challenge to medicine, and the questions researchers are asking are the same ones people with diabetes or those with a family history of the disease are wondering about. Persons with diabetes are worried about their family members—brothers, sisters, parents—getting diabetes, and parents are especially concerned about transmitting it to their children.

The genetics of diabetes is very complicated, much more so than we thought 10 years ago. At that time, for instance, we thought that if an identical twin got diabetes, the other would always develop it as well; or if both parents had diabetes, then all their children would also get it. Clinical studies have not substantiated this. At the Joslin Clinic, where follow-up studies have been going on for as long as 20 years, they've found that if an identical twin develops Type I, insulin-dependent diabetes, there may be only a 50% chance that the other twin will develop diabetes as well. And if both parents have diabetes, the children may stand less than a 50% chance of developing diabetes requiring treatment.

Another study that was rather surprising was reported in *The New England Journal of Medicine* (311:149, 1984) where it was shown that a father may be more likely to transmit diabetes to his children than a mother. This is very perplexing, I for one might think that a mother who has had diabetes since childhood and during her pregnancy would be likely to transmit diabetes to her children. But that was not found to be the case.

In my own practice I have seen over 20,000 patients, the hereditary aspects of diabetes are definitely not clear. In my own case, for instance, I am one of five brothers, and both my father and mother come from families with five children. Between us, my brothers and I have 6 children. Yet I am the only one in our large family who has diabetes. On the other hand, there are extended families with no previous history of diabetes where diabetes then appears in two or three children of the same parents. Then there are some extended families where there is a much greater incidence. This tend to be more common in Type II non-insulin-dependent diabetes. There are several families in my practice where as many as four or five brothers and/or sisters have diabetes, especially when the onset is over the age of forty. This is more true in families where there is a higher incidence of obesity, since obesity is likely to contribute to the diabetes. In other families there were a grandfather, father and son all with diabetes.

So from the practical standpoint, what does all this confusing information mean? It means that there is no simple answer. We need to work on human genes to see which ones could be involved in transmitting diabetes. Theoretically, if we could identify the persons who may be susceptible to developing diabetes, we could work on the preventive aspects. For example, if a person has the gene or genes for diabetes, we might check to see if he or she is developing beta cell or insulin antibodies. If these antibodies are present, then maybe we can use medications (see Chapter 30, "Research: The Quest for a Cure") to limit further antibody production and thereby ward off their tendencies to destroy beta cells.

In the case of Type II non-insulin-dependent diabetes (where the heredity transmission is even greater than in Type I insulin-dependent diabetes), if we could identify whether a family member has definitely inherited the gene, then he or she could be watched more closely for the development of diabetes. Remember, diabetes can be present silently for a number of years in many people before it manifests itself. Maybe the diagnosis isn't made until it's already advanced and complications have developed. So, if the tendency for diabetes (i.e., the genetic trait) can be discovered and the diabetes diagnosed earlier, then treatment can be started earlier and complications forestalled.

The above sounds good, but unfortunately the study of genes is not so easy; there are an estimated 50,000 human genes. In addition, there may be more than one of them that's responsible for the development of diabetes. At this point therefore genetic studies are available at special research centers only and are not available for the average person.

In summary then, the hereditary transmission of diabetes is known to be important in some more than others. But we have not been able to identify all the genes that are responsible, since there are so many. I would therefore recommend that people who have a strong family history of Type II diabetes should eat right, and keep slim and physically active in the hope of preventing diabetes. Although there are some genetic studies of Type I diabetes, there's nothing absolute that might help us now to identify those who may someday get it. Until we have more information, it's hard to advise family members on what the risks are for brothers and sisters or for children of developing diabetes.

Will diabetes prevent a person from leading a satisfying and successful life? I've saved this question for last because it's perhaps the greatest fear that a person has when he first develops diabetes. I had the same fear myself just after I

developed diabetes and was beginning my career in medicine. I thought all my goals for becoming a doctor would be
thwarted. What a mistaken fear that, was! It has been 28 years
since then, during which time my life has blossomed bounti-
fully. I'm able to spend long hours giving care to my patients,
with my greatest reward in being able to see them through
their illness. Not only has my medical career been satisfying,
but so has my family life with four healthy and energetic
children who are launching careers of their own now.

I've been able to retain my athletic skills with long-
distance running and local championship tennis. I spend
time cultivating flower and vegetable gardens, and finally,
I've been able to use my "secret talent" to become a respected
writer, the author of several well-received books that have
been acknowledged by professional and lay people alike.
Need I say more? Well, I should say that there are and have
been many people like me who haven't let diabetes hinder
their careers. To name a few: Menachem Begin, former prime
minister of Israel; Tim Belknap, Mr. Universe 1985; Jack
Benny, comedian; Paul Cezanne, artist; Bobby Clarke, hockey
player; Thomas Edison, inventor; Bill Gullickson, base ball
player; Howard Hughes, industrialist; Jim "Catfish" Hunter,
base ball player; Peggy Lee, singer; Mary Tyler Moore, actress;
Elvis Presley, singer, actor; Jackie Robinson, baseball player;
Bill Talbert, tennis player; H. G. Wells, author. The list goes
on and on. The one thing always to remember is that with
diabetes you too can have a happy, productive and richly
rewarding life.

Finally, I am glad to say that since my health has held up
so well I have been able to meet up with one of the most
beautiful women in the world, Becky. Wow, how lucky I am
to be able to share my life and love with her. She is a true
soulmate.

32

Recommended Readings

Below is a brief list of additional educational material that can provide the latest information about diabetes, nutrition, and exercise. This list is greatly abbreviated and you should check the bookstore and library for the many other excellent books that can help you understand and manage your diabetes.

Diabetes Forecast—A bimonthly publication containing up-to-date diabetes information, including current theories about diabetes, dietary information, short biographies of famous people with diabetes or people who have lived many years with diabetes, as well as other helpful material. It can be obtained through the American Diabetes Association (1660 Duke Street, Alexandria, VA 22314).

The Pritikin Program for Diet and Exercise, by Nathan Pritikin and Patrick M. McGrady, Jr., published in 1979 by Grosset & Dunlop; paperback from Bantam Books. This book is a very controversial best-seller that has caused quite a stir in the medical community because of its drastic dietary recommendations. It proposes that 80% of the calories in one's daily diet should be in the form of high-fiber carbohydrates and less than 20% of the caloric intake should be in the form of protein and fat. Although there has been no definitive empirical proof that such a diet will indeed prolong the life span or prevent arteriosclerosis, this book makes some excellent nutritional points. It emphasizes the benefit of exercise in conjunction with proper diet, and there is no doubt that the Pritikin program can help control high blood pressure as well as diabetes in some people. People with brittle diabetes may have a hard time controlling their diabetes with so many carbohydrates, particularly fruits.

The Sports Medicine Book, by Gabe Mirkin, M.D., and Marshall Hoffman, published in 1978 by Little, Brown. Dr. Mirkin offers some provoking ideas about exercise and nutrition. Especially interesting is his discussion on the value of vitamins. He discusses programs for "peak" performance and suggests how injuries can be prevented and managed. This book may be very helpful to the sportsminded diabetes person, even though it is not written specifically for the person with diabetes.

Diabetes Sports and Exercise Book, by Claudia Graham, Ph.D., C.D.E., June Biermann and Barbara Toohey, 1995. This a totally new, up-dated version of our popular 1977 book, which was based on the sports experiences of 168 exercise enthusiasts with diabetes. They were the only people who could give help and counsel at that time, since medical science did not recognize the importance of exercise for diabetes control and well-being. This 1995 edition contains all the new scientific and technical information about exercising with diabetes – and that's a lot of information!

The Diabetic's Sports and Exercise Book, by June Biermann and Barbara Toohey, published in 1977 by J.B. Lippincott. This is the first comprehensive book for the person with diabetes who exercises. It emphasizes the effectiveness of exercise in controlling diabetes, and in lowering the insulin requirements for the insulin-dependent person with diabetes. The book is especially inspirational for the weight-conscious person with diabetes.

Managing Your Gestational Diabetes, by Lois Jovanovic-Peterson, M.D. with Morton B. Stone, 1994. Dr. Jovanovic-Peterson is one of the country's leading authorities on gestational diabetes(a temporary form of diabetes that appears during pregnancy). This book guides you through the steps to control your diabetes and reduce risks to yourself and your baby. Essential reading for mothers-to-be who develop this form of diabetes.

The Diabetic's Total Health Book, by June Biermann and Barbara Toohey, published in 1980 by J. P. Tarcher (9110 Sunset Boulevard, Los Angeles, CA 90069). Another very readable and thorough book by Biermann and Toohey.

Vegetarian Cooking for People with Diabetes, by Patricia LaShane, 1994. Over 100 true vegan recipes with dairy products or eggs, emphasizing low-fat cooking. Soy mild used for protein, along with nuts, grains and legumes (beans, lentils, garban-zos, soybeans, etc.). Sweeteners amounts of blackstrap molasses or honey. No white flour or sugar.

The Calculating Cook, by Jeanne Jones, published by 101 Productions (79 Liberty Street, San Francisco, CA 94110). This excellent hook shows how to create low-calorie gourmet meals. It also describes how food can be made in quantity and then preserved, which is helpful to the individual who is hard-pressed for time.

The Joslin Diabetes Gourmet Cookbook, by Bonnie Polin & Frances Giedt, 1993. Created under the aegis of the Joslin Clinic, this is a glorious collection of over 530 fabulous recipes for people with diabetes and cardiovascular problems (low in fat, cholesterol, sugar and salt). Both authors have diabetes and a passion for good food.

Joslin Diabetes Manual, edited by Leo J. Krall, 11th edition, published in 1978 by Lea & Febiger. This comprehensive work is written by physicians and other professionals of the Joslin Clinic, where, for over 60 years, diabetes has been studied more intensely than in any other place in the world.

Diabetes: A Practical New Guide to Healthy Living, by .James W. Anderson, M.D., published in 1981 by Arco (219 Park Avenue

South, New York, NY10003). Dr. James W. Anderson, a renowned expert in the diabetes field, outlines his highly successful ways of treating diabetes with special emphasis on how to incorporate high-fiber carbohydrate to help reduce the need for insulin in many patients as well as lower their cholesterol and blood fat levels.

Fit or Fat Target Diet, by Covert Bailey, published in 1984 by Houghton Mifflin. This is really not just another diet book, but an approach to eating. I recommend it for many people who can't control their impulse to overeat. They will succeed more often.

The Fit or Fat Woman, by Covert Bailey and LEa Bishop, 1989. This book applies Bailey's successful weight loss strategy to women, acknowledging that "women have more trouble with fat than men." The focus of this program is to lower your body's percentage of fat and increase its percentage of muscle. The goal is to reduce your body to a healthy level of 19 to 22% fat.

The New Fit or Fat?, by Covert Bailey, 1991. The essential message of this well researched, breakthrough book is that overweight people should concentrate on losing body fat, not pounds.

Lean & Mean: The No Hassle, Life-Extending Weight Loss Program for Men, by Morton Shaevitz, 1993. Recommendations are decrease dietary fat, increase complex carbohydrates, limit alcohol and exercise 45 minutes to an hour five or six days a week. Crammed with good strategies for eating at convention and meetings, in restaurants and on airplanes. *Not* a diet, but a good way of life for life.

Protein Power, by Michael Eades, M.D. and Mary Dan Eades, M.D., 1996. This eye-opening, scientifically convincing book describes a new dietary approach to managing obesity, Type II diabetes, heart disease, high blood pressure and elevated cholesterol. It is a complete turnaround from the nutritional establishment's current high-carbohydrate, low-fat theories.

The Type II Diabetes Diet Book, by Calvin Ezrin, M.D. and Robert E. Kowalski, 1995. Dr. Ezrin, an eminent endocrinologist, is one of the pioneers in using a low carbohydrate diet for weight loss. His new book is directed to Type II's who are at least 20% overweight. His research and clinical experience have taught him that such people suffer from an identifiable hormonal disorder called "hyperinsulinism."

Diabetes, Research for Health and Freedom, by Dorothea Sims, published in 1984, by C.V. Moseby (11830 Westline Industrial Dr., St. Louis, MO 63146). Nicely written book by someone who can give plenty of answers, having had diabetes for over 30 years. I definitely like the tone of this book. *The Diabetic Woman,* by Lois Jovanovic, M.D., June Biermann and Barbara Toohey, published in 1987 by Jeremy P. Tarcher, Inc. (Los Angeles, CA). An excellent book that discusses how a woman can effectively manage diabetes in all phases of her life.

The Diabetic Man, by Peter A. Lodewick, M.D., June Biermann and Barbara Toohey published by Lowell House, Los Angeles, 1992. The guide to health and success in all areas of a man's life: career, sports, travel, sex, impotence, relationships, and everything else. Includes advice, empathy and support for those with a man with diabetes in their lives and for parents of a son with diabetes.

The Diabetic Woman, by Lois Jovanovic-Peterson, M.D., June Biermann and Barbara Toohey, 1987. The only book to focus on how women can deal with diabetes-related problems at the different ages and stages of their lives. Here is medical advice and support and understanding as well as realistic coping methods for the complex concerns of today's woman. Diabetes Self Management (P.O. Box 851, Farmingdale, NY 11737). A bimonthly publication giving a world of diabetes practical tidbits on self care.

Diabetes: A Practical New Guide to Healthy Living, by James Anderson, M.D., 1981. This book delivers a message that person with diabetes can take control of their own diabetes and lead rewarding lives through proper diet and exercise.

The Diabetic's Book: All Your Questions Answered, by June Biermann and Barbara Toohey, 3rd edition 1994. The classic first book to read when you're diagnosed person with diabetes.

Diabetic's Total Health Book, by June Biermann and Barbara Toohey, 3rd edition 1992. This is the book that proves you can have diabetes yet be the picture of health, leading a vital, productive, happy life. How to focus on health rather than on disease and how to achieve a strong body, a tranquil mind and a blithe spirit.

The Peripatetic Diabetic, by June Biermann and Barbara Toohey, 1984. Our first and most personal and humorous diabetes book. Tells how you feel when you're diagnosed, how to overcome your initial fear and despair and go on to a joyful and exciting life.

The Diabetes Self-Care Method, by Charles Peterson, M.D. and Lois Jovanovic-Peterson, M.D., 1990, An innovative, success-ful program by two of the foremost endocrinologists of the U.S. (one has diabetes). Focuses on normalizing blood sugar through self-testing and insulin adjustment to give you a free and flexible lifestyle. Exactly the kind of self-care the DCCT recommends for avoiding complications.

Stop the Rollercoaster, by John Walsh, PA, CDE, Ruth Roberts, and Lois Jovanovic-Peterson, M.D., 1995. If you have inexplic-able blood sugar climbs and plunges, help is here! This timely manual, written by three highly experienced professionals – two with insulin-dependent diabetes – is for all Type I's and the 40% of Type II's who use insulin. Features Flexible Insulin Therapy, the proven-successful method of using multiple injections to mimic the body's way of maintaining normal blood sugar, thereby giving you a more normal, flexible and healthy lifestyle and a complication-free future.

The Glucograph Method of Normalizing Blood Sugar, by Richard K. Bernstein, M.D., published in 1981 by Jeremy P. Tarcher, Inc. (Los Angeles, CA). A very methodical approach to treating Type I diabetes. Dr. Bernstein feels that if all insulin-dependent people followed his suggestions, they would keep their blood sugars completely normal. (His approach is applicable to those who are willing to do five to seven blood sugars per day.) His high fat diet is against the mainstream of current thought, which advocates low fat, and high fiber and carbohydrate.

Resources

American Diabetes Association
1660 Duke Street
Alexandria, VA 22314

Membership includes subscription to the informative Diabetes Forecast, as well as the opportunity to join local chapters, scattered throughout the country, which run frequent meetings to discuss and seek answers to the problems of diabetes.

HCF Diabetes Foundation
Box 22124
Lexington, KY 40522

Founded by James W. Anderson, M.D., a pioneer in the high-fiber complex carbohydrate diet to control diabetes and cholesterol. Has newsletter and provides educational material to help keep the individual with diabetes in good control.

Juvenile Diabetes Foundation International
Executive Office
60 Madison Avenue
New York, NY 10010

An energetic voluntary organization originally formed to find the answers to diabetes through research but which along the way has added education and support groups to aid in the fight against diabetes.

The Sugar Free Center, Inc.
13715 Burbank Boulevard
Box 114
Van Nuys, CA 91408

Founded by June Biermann and Barbara Toohey, both prolific diabetes authors, to allow customers to secure diabetes literature and materials (insulin, syringes, blood sugar testing apparatus, etc.) at reasonable prices.

Diabetic Reader
Prana* Publications & Paraphernalia
5623 Matilija Avenue
Van Nuys, CA 91401
1(800) 735-7726

The Diabetic Reader is a production of June Biermann and Barbara Toohey.

Diabetes Interview
3715 Balboa Street
San Francisco, CA 94121

The Diabetes Care Center
Peter A. Lodewick
700 18th Street, South, Suite 403
Birmingham, Ala. 35233

Index

Banik, Allen E., Dr., 137
Banting, Frederick G., Dr., 4
Basal Bolus System, 65-66
Baxter Health Care
  System, 34
Begin, Menachem, 256
Belknap, Tim, 51, 256
Benign retinopathy, 199
Benny, Jack,256
Berenstein Diet, 94-95
Berenstein, Richard, Dr., 94
Best, Charles H., Dr., 4
Beta cells, 4, 77, 230, 240-242
Beta-hydroxybutyrate, 81
Biermann, June, 67
Big Wolf Lake, 135
Biocontrol Technology, 35
BioDynamics, 43
Birth. See Pregnancy
  and birth
Bladder, 204
Blindness. See Eye
  complications
Blisters. See Corns and
  calluses
Blood pressure, 204-205
Blood sugar. See glucose
  headings; Hypoglycemia;
  Insulin; Sugar; Tests,
  diabetes
Blood sugar testing. See
  Glycohemoglobin mea
  surement; Home
  monitoring, blood sugar;
  tests, diabetes
Blood vessels, large, 205-206
Body cream. See Creams
Boehringer Mannheim

Diagnostics, 34
Books on diabetes, 258-264
Borderline Diabetes, 10
Bread, 2, 96, 116-117, 121
Breast-feeding, 187
Brittle diabetes
  Berenstein diet and, 94-95
  calories and, 94-96
  carbohydrates and, 94-96
  causes, 86-91
  defined, 86
  dental care and, 161
  diabetes neuropathy
  and, 93
  insulin and, 86
  management of, 86-92
  somoygi effect and, 91-92
Butazolidin, 49

C

Calcium, 135, 179
Calluses. See Corns and
  calluses
Calories, 141
  in alcohol, 217-219
  defined, 104
  effects on diabetes control,
  95-96
  exercise expended in,
  153-154
  individual needs, 103
  pregnancy, recommend
  ed, 183
  weight loss and, 142
Candida. See Yeast infection.
Carbohydrates, 93-94, 105,
  146-147

Ketones, 81
Ketonuria, 185
Ketosis, 2. See Ketoacidosis.
Ketostix, 43
Kidneys, 38, 203-204
Kussmaul breathing, 81

L

Landers, Ann, 190
Landone, Brown, M.D., 138
Laser treatment, 200-201
Latent chemical diabetes, 7
LeanLine, 250
Lee, Peggy, 256
Legs, 171, 205. See also
    Foot Care.
Lifescan, Inc., 35
Lipoprotein, 106
Lomotil, 216
Loprox, 174
Low blood sugar. See
    Hypoglycemia.
Low density lipoprotein
    (LDL), 107
Lupus, 164
Lys-Pro, 231-232

M

Meat, 114, 118-119
Medication. See Pills.
Medi-Jector Lab/Medi-
    Jector II, 66-67
Menstruation and
    menopause, 177-179
Merthiolate, 173
Metaphen, 173

Meters. See Home
    monitoring.
Metoclopramide, 205
Microaneurysms, 199
Micronase, 46, 76
Micro Pore, 173
Miles Laboratories, 34
Milk, 114, 126, 146
Monilia, 18, 168
Monounsaturated fat, 106
Moore, Mary Tyler, 256
Mumps, 228-229

N

Nasal spray, 249
National Eye Institute, 201
National Geographic, 138
National Institutes of Health
    (NIH), 6, 223, 229, 249
Nervous system, 203-204
Neuritis, 204, 218
Neuropathy, 168, 172, 190,
203
*The New England Journal of
Medicine*, 144, 249, 253
Nicotinic acid, 47-48
Non-insulin-dependent
    diabetes
    and brittle diabetes,242-
243
    characteristics, 5-9
    diet for, 16, 131-132
    exercise and, 156-157
    menses and, 178-179
    research advances, 242-
243
    symptoms, 16

urine testing for, 38
Novolin Prefill™, 57, 239-240
NovoPen, 56-57, 67, 239
Notkins, Abner L., Dr., 229
Novo-Nordisk Research
    Labs, 56, 231, 240
Nursing. See Breast-feeding.
Nutrient, 105
Nuts, 127, 142

O

Obesity, 20
    see also Weight loss
Older people, diabetes and, 5
One Touch II, 34
Oral hypoglycemic agents.
    See Pills; specific drug
    names
Orange Medical Instruments,
    35
Orinase, 44, 46, 76
Osbon Medical Systems, 191
Osteoporosis, 179
Overeaters Anonymous, 142,
    250
Overt diabetes, 10

P

Pancreas
    glucagon and, 77
    insulin and, 2-3, 20
    transplantation, 240-241
Paralysis, 205
Papaverine, 191
Pauling, Linus, Dr., 108
Peanuts, 127

Pectin, 108
Penile Nocturnal Tumescence
    Study, 190
Penile prosthesis, 191
Penlet, 33
Pen Pump, 238-239
Performance Medical, 191
Period, menstrual, 177-178
Periodontal disease, 161
Periodontist, 164
Pills, 44-48
    See also specific names.
Plaque, 164-165
Podiatrist, 173
Polyunsaturated fat, 106
Poor circulation, 172
Post-T-Vac, Inc., 191
Postprandial blood sugar test,
    25
Powers, Pete, 149
Precijet, 67
Prediabetes, 9-10
Pregnancy and birth
    breast-feeding, 187
    complications, 182-183
    delivery, 184-185
    diabetes control after, 186
    on control, 221
    diabetes developed
        during, 19, 182
    diabetes prior to, 182-185
    diabetes signs in, 19
    diet, 184
    fetal monitoring, 185
    home monitoring
        during, 31
    in insulin-dependent
        woman, 183

ABOUT THE AUTHOR

PETER A. LODEWICK, M.D., is currently Medical Director of the Diabetes Care Center, located at The Eye Foundation Hospital in Birmingham, Alabama.

Dr. Lodewick received his medical training at the Boston University School of Medicine, and later was the recipient of a fellowship from the Joslin Diabetes Center in Boston. He enjoys writing, gardening and tennis in addition to his medical responsibilities of providing good care to people with diabetes.

If you seek information or consultation regarding any information in this book, Dr. Lodewick can be contacted by writing .

Peter A. Lodewick, M.D.
P.O. Box 550160
Birmingham, Alabama 35205

Southern Publishers Group
147 Corporate Way
Pelham, AL 35124
Toll Free Number: 1-800-628-0903

TO ORDER ADDITIONAL COPIES

Please send me ___ copies of "A Diabetic Doctor Looks At Diabetes - His and Yours" at a cost of $14.95 plus $2.50 Shipping and Handling.

Please send me ____ copies of "The Diabetic Man" at a cost of $15.95 plus $2.50 Shipping and Handling.

Please send me ____ copies of "Diabetes and Distilled Water" at a cost of $1.95 plus $2.50 Shipping and Handling.

Enclosed is my check in the amount of $ _____

Please charge to my MasterCard or Visa Account:

Account #_____

Exp. _____   MC Interbank #_____

Authorized Signature_____

Ship to: _____

_____

Name _____

Institution (if applicable)_____

Street_____

City _____ State _____ Zip_____

Southern Publishers Group
147 Corporate Way